"BOSS Series"

Physiology

"BOSS Series"
Physiology

O.P. Tandon
MD, FIC, MNAMS, FAMS, FIABS

Professor and Head
Department of Physiology
University College of Medical Sciences
(University of Delhi) and
GTB Hospital, Dilshad Garden
Delhi-110095

PEEPEE
PUBLISHERS AND DISTRIBUTORS (P) LTD.

"BOSS Series" Physiology

Published by
Pawaninder P. Vij
Peepee Publishers and Distributors (P) Ltd.
Head Office: 160, Shakti Vihar, Pitam Pura
New Delhi-110 034
Corporate Office: 7/31, Ansari Road, Daryaganj
Post Box-7243
New Delhi-110002 (India)
Ph: 55195868, 9811156083
e-mail: peepee160@yahoo.co.in
e-mail: peepee160@rediffmail.com
www.peepeepub.com

First Edition: **2005**

ISBN: 81-88867-54-3

Printed at
Lordson, C-5/19, Rana Pratap Bagh, Delhi-110 007

To
The students
who toil so hard,
lead stressful life
to achieve their goals

Preface

Physiology is a vast, everexpanding subject. It is almost impossible to remain update with all the facts, when new ones are being added all the time. It is in this context, the author felt the need for a small book as a ready reckoner in physiology. This book is based on facts in basic, systemic and applied physiology, which will not only update the knowledge of physiology with its latest developments but also serve as a quick revision before the examination (viz viva voce, practicals, tutorials, SSQs, and MCQ's for various entrance exams)—A MUST FOR ALL THE STUDENTS.

Last minute 'check' and confirmation of answers before the exam builds up student's confidence and improves his performance and score. This book will be a boon to the students of physiology appearing in MBBS, BDS, B Pharma, B PTH, B OTH, MSc, MD and various entrance and competitive examinations.

The author is thankful to Mr Pawaninder Pal Vij for publishing this book.

Suggestions to improve the book are welcome.

O.P. Tandon

Contents

Chapter One

General Physiology

a. Principles of Organisation

- **Cell** is a simple, basic, structural and functional **unit** of living being.
- Cell **differentiation** results in formation of **four categories** of specialized cells.
  a. **Muscle cells** generate mechanical activities that produce **force** and **movement**.
  b. **Nerve cells** initiate and conduct **electrical signals**.
  c. **Epithelial cells** selectively **secrete** and **absorb** ions and **organic molecules**.
  d. **Connective tissue** cells connect, anchor and **support** the structures of the body.
- Specialized cells **associate** with similar cells to form **tissues** i.e. muscle tissue, nerve tissue, epithelial tissue and connective tissue.
- **Organs** are composed of the **four kind** of **tissues** arranged in various **proportions** and **patterns**.
- Many organs contain multiple **small and similar** functional **units**.
- The **extracellular fluid** surrounding a cell is the cell's **internal environment**.
- **Maintenance** of internal environment (**milieu interior**) **constant** and stable is usually referred to as **homeostasis**.
- The **function** of **organ systems** of the body is to maintain the **internal environment** relatively constant.

- Each cell performs the basic cellular processes required to maintain its **own integrity** plus **specialised** activities that help **maintain** the **internal environment** relatively constant—**homeostasis**.
- The extracellular fluid is **composed** of blood **plasma** and the fluid between cells—**interstitial fluid**.
- Of the extra cellular fluid, **80%** is **interstitial fluid** and **20% plasma**.
- Interstitial fluid (80%) and plasma (20%) have essentially **same composition** except that **plasma** contains much higher concentration of **protein**.
- Extracellular fluid **differs** markedly in composition from the fluid inside cells—intracellular fluid.

b. Chemical Composition of Body

- **Atoms** are composed of three subatomic particles; positive protons, neutral **neutrons** (both located in **nucleus**) and negative **electrons** revolving around the nucleus.
- The atomic **number** is the number of **protons** in the **nucleus** of atom, but since atom is electrically neutral, it is also equal to **number** of **electrons**.
- The atomic **mass** is an atom's mass **relative** to that of a **carbon-12,** atom. It is approximately equal to number of **protons + neutrons**.
- **One gram** atomic **mass** is the number of grams of an element equal to its **atomic mass**.
- **Molecules** are formed by linking **atoms together. Covalent bond** is formed when two atoms **share** a **pair of electrons** between them.
- Each type of atom can form a characteristic number of covalent bonds: **Hydrogen 1, oxygen 2, nitrogen 3** and **carbon 4**.
- Molecules have characteristic **shapes** that can be altered within limits by the **rotation** of their atoms around **covalent bonds**.

- When an **atom gains** or **loses** one or **more electrons**, it acquires a **net electronic charge** and becomes an **ion**.
- In **polar** covalent bonds, one atom attracts the bonding electrons more than does the other atoms.
- **Water**, a **polar molecule**, is attracted to other water molecule by **hydrogen bond**.
- **Substances** dissolved in a liquid are **solutes** and the **liquid** in which they are **dissolved** is the **solvent**.
- **Water** is the most **abundant** solvent in the **body**.
- The **molecular mass** of a molecule is the **sum** of the **atomic** masses of all its atoms.
- **One gram molecule** of any substance contains **6.02×10^{23} molecules (Avogadros number).**
- Substances that **release** a **hydrogen ion** in solution are called **acids**. Those that **accept** hydrogen ion are **bases**.
- The **acidity** of a solution is determined by its **free hydrogen ion** concentration, the **greater it is the greater acidity**.
- The **pH** of a solution is the **negative log of the hydrogen ion** concentration, as the **acidity** of a solution **increases**, the **pH decreases**.
- **Pure water** has pH of **7.0** (neutral).
- **Carbohydrates** are composed of **carbon**, **hydrogen** and **oxygen** in proportions C_{12} $(H_2O)n$.
- The presence of **polar** hydroxyl groups makes carbohydrates **soluble** in water.
- The most abundant **monosaccharide** in the body is **glucose** which is **stored** in cells in form of **glycogen**.
- **Lipids** (fats) lack polar and **ionized groups**, a characteristic that makes them **insoluble** in water.
- **Triglycerides** are formed when **fatty acids** are **linked** to each of the three **hydroxyl** groups in **glycerol**.
- **Steroids** are composed of **four interconnected rings** often containing a few polar **hydroxyl groups**.

- **Proteins** macromolecules are composed primarily of **carbon**, **hydrogen**, **oxygen** and **nitrogen** and are **polymers** of **amino acids**.
- The primary structure of **polypeptide** chain is determined by **number** of **amino acids** in **sequence** and the **type of amino** acid at each position.
- **Nucleic acids** are responsible for the **storage, expression**, and **transmission of genetic** information.
- Nucleic acids are **polymers** of **nucleotides**, each containing a **phosphate group**, a **sugar** and **a ring of carbon** and **nitrogen atoms** known as **base**.
- **DNA** consists of **two chains** of **nucleotides**, coiled around each other in a **double helix**.
- The chains are held together by **hydrogen bonds** between **purine** and **pyrimidine** bases in the two chains.
- **Base pairing** in **DNA** always occurs between **guanine, cytosine** and **adenine-thymine**.
- **RNA** consists of **single chain** of **nucleotides**, containing the **sugar ribose** and **three** of the **four bases** found in **DNA**. The fourth base is **pyrimidine uracil** rather than thymine. Uracil **base-pairs** with **adenosine**.
- **DNA stores genetic information** whereas **RNA** is involved in **decoding** it into instruction for linking together **amino acids** to form **proteins**.

Chapter Two

Cell Physiology

- Every **cell** has **membrane** and **nonmembrane** bound particles and filaments called cellular **organelle**.
- Cell **membrane** consists of a **bimolecular lipid layer**, mainly phospholipids in which **proteins** are embedded.
- The lipid layer **prevents** the **movement** of most **molecules** through the membrane while the **proteins** provide **pathway** for the **selective entry** of substances.
- **Three** types of **membrane junctions** link **adjacent cells**.
  a. **Desmosomes** link cells that are subject to considerable **stretching**.
  b. **Tight junctions** found primarily in **epithelial cells**, limit the passage of molecules through extracellular space between the cells.
  c. **Gap junction** form **channels** between cytoplasm of adjacent cells.
- Cell **organelle** and their **functions**.
  a. The **nucleus** transmits and expresses **genetic information**.
  b. The **nucleolus** is the **site** at which **ribosomes** are formed.
  c. **Granular** endoplasmic **reticulum** is primarily involved in the **packaging** of proteins that are to be **secreted** from the cells.
  d. **A granular** endoplasmic reticulum is tubular, lacks ribosomes and is site of **lipid formation**.
  e. Ribosomes composed of **RNA** and protein are the site of proteins synthesis.

f. **Mitochondria** are the major sites for **energy transformed** in form of ATP. they are the power house of the cell factory.
g. **Lysosomes** digest the particulate matter which **enters** the cell.
h. **Peroxisomes** break down certain **toxic products** formed from **oxygen**.

- **Four** types of **filaments** form **cytoskeleton** of the cell: They are **microfilaments, intermediate filaments, muscle thick filaments** and **microtubules**.
- Using bacterial **enzymes, segment** of **DNA** can be **cut** from DNA of **one organism** and **inserted** into DNA of **another organism** to form **recombinant DNA** which will then **direct** the **synthesis of proteins, coded by** donor **DNA** in the **host organism**.
- **Cancer cells** are characterised by their **capacity** for **unlimited multiplication** and ability to **metastasise** to other parts of body.
- **Mutation** of certain **growth regulating genes** into **oncogenes** can **transform** normal cell to a **cancer cell**.
- **More than** one **mutation** may be necessary to cause this **transformation** to **cancer cell**.
- In all cells, **energy** is transferred from **catabolism** of **fuel molecules** to **ATP. Hydrolysis** of **ATP** to **ADP and P_1** then transfer the **energy** to cell function.
- **ATP** is formed from **oxidative phosphorylation** and **substrate phosphorylation**.
- The **enzymes** for **oxidative phophorilation** are located on the **inner membrane** of **mitochondria**.
- The end products of **aerobic glycolysis** are **ATP** and **pyruvic acid** and those of **anaerobic glycolysis** are **ATP** and **lactic acid**.
- The majority of the **hydrogen** atoms used in **oxidative phosphorylation** are derived from reaction in the **Kreb's cycle**, whose **enzymes** are located in the **matrix** of the **mitochondria**.

- **Acetyl CoA** is the **major substrate** entering the **Kreb's cycle**.
- Under **aerobic conditions 38 molecules** of **ATP** can be **formed** from **1 molecule** of **glucose**: **34 ATP** can be formed from **oxidative phosphorilation from coenzyme-2H, 2ATP** by **glycolysis** and **2 ATP** by **substrate phosphorylation** in **Kreb's cycle**.
- Under **anaerobic** condition, **2 mols** of **ATP** are formed from **1 mol** of **glucose**.
- About **40%** of chemical energy in **glucose** can be transferred to **ATP** under **aerobic conditions**, the rest appears as heat.
- **Glucose** can be **synthesised** from some **amino acids** and **from lactic** acid and glycerol (Neoglucogenesis). **Fatty acids cannot** be used for this purpose.
- Fat **stored** in **adipose tissue**, provides about **80%** of the **stored fuel** in body.
- **Fatty acids** are broken down in the **mitochondrial inner compartment** by **beta oxidation**.
- The amount of **ATP** formed by **breakdown** of 1 **gram of fat** is about **2½ times greater** than the **ATP** released from **1 gm of glucose**.
- **Fatty acids** are **synthesised** from acetyl CoA by enzymes **located** in **cytosol** and are linked to **glycerophosphate** to form **triglycerols** by **enzymes** in the **smooth endoplasmic reticulum**.
- Proteins are **broken** down into **amino acids** by **protease**.
- **Amino** groups of protein are **removed** by:
  a. Oxidative **deamination** giving rise to **ammonia.**
  b. **Transamination** in which amino groups is transferred to a **keto acid** to form new **amino acid**.
- The **ammonia** formed by oxidative **deamination** is converted into **urea** in **liver** and excreted in **urine** by kidney.

a. Transport Functions of Plasma Membranes

- **Secretion:** Cells release products of their synthesis into extracellular space by means of secretion.
- **Lipid soluble materials** synthesized by cells, like steroid hormones, prostaglandin are secreted through **diffusion** across the cell membrane.
- **Small water soluble** molecules and macromolecules are secreted into extracellular space by **exocytosis**.
- **Exocytosis** is the process in which vesicles containing secretory products fuse with cell membrane to release their contents.
- **Types** of secretory processes are two:
  a. **Constituted secretion**, which operates continuously in the cell in order to maintain integrity of plasma membrane, thus provides a mean of inserting proteins into plasma membrane (repairs the wear and tear).
  b. **Regulated secretion**, which occurs in response to specific signals. The principal signal for regulated secretion is a rise in intracellular calcium.
- **Endocytosis** is the process of retrieval of the vesicular membrane fused with plasma membrane during exocytosis. Some cells take up large proteins from extracellular fluid by **receptor mediated endocytosis**.
- **Phagocytosis** (Phagos -eat, cytose - cell)—Specialised cells (Reticulo endothelial, macrophages, leukocytes) engulf foreign particles and cell debris by a process, called phagocytosis.
- **Gases**, as they are lipid soluble, readily pass through the lipid bilayer plasma membrane down their concentration gradient by **passive transport** (Diffusion).
- **Ions** and **other polar molecules**, unlike gases cannot diffuse through lipid bilayer membrane but cross it via the **aqueous pore** of **channel**

proteins or are transported across the plasma membrane by **carrier proteins**.

- **Active transport**—For a substance to be accumulated against its **electrochemical gradient, energy** must be expended. In active transport energy is provided by the hydrolysis of **ATP** (i.e. sodium pump) or by coupling the movement of one substance against its electrochemical gradient to the movement of another down its electrochemical gradient—this is **secondary active transport**. The sodium dependent uptake of glucose by the enterocytes is one example (**symport**).
- **Intracellular cations**—The major intracellular cation is K^+.
- **Extracellular cations**—Sodium is the principal extracellular cation along with chloride which is anion.
- The **sodium pump** is an example of ATP driven active transport.
- **Na^+–H^+ exchange,** Na–Ca^{++} exchange are examples of secondary active transport. In both their transports, energy is provided by the sodium gradient generated by the sodium pump.
- **Main functions** of sodium pump which is a **carrier protein** and not ion channel, are:
  a. Exchange intracellular Na^+ for extracellular K^+.
  b. Directly links Na^+ efflux with K^+ influx.
  c. Is important for maintaining a constant cell volume.
  d. It requires ATP and thus can be inhibited by metabolic poisons.
- **The resting membrane potential,** is a potential difference across the resting cell membrane of excitable tissue. Its value for **skeletal muscle** is closer to the K+ equilibrium potential and **is –90 mV**.
- The resting membrane potential is **determined by K+ gradient** because there are many more **open K+ channels** than **Na^+ channels.** Conse-

quently resting membrane potential is close to **potassium equilibrium potential**.

b. Principles of Cell Signalling

- **Hormones** are secreted by **endocrine glands** into the blood stream to act on cells at **a distance**.
- **Hormones** are **chemical signals** secreted by **specialised glands having no ducts**.
- **Paracrine factors** are **signals** which act on **surrounding cells**.
- **Nitric oxide** and **prostaglandins** are examples of **paracrine signalling molecules.**
- **Calcium** and **cyclic AMP** are both **intracellular mediators** but **cyclic AMP** can **spread** from **cell to cell** via **gap junctions**.
- Many receptors are **membrane proteins** or **membrane bound enzymes** but some are **intra-cellular proteins** (e.g. **steroid hormone receptors**).
- **Receptors** may activate **ion channels directly** but some receptors are **protein kinase** that are activated when they **bind** their **ligand**.
- Many **receptors activate G-protein** and thereby **modulate** the levels of **second messengers.**
- **Prostaglandins** are **metabolites of arachidonic** acid that is derived from **membrane phos-pholipids** by the **action of phospholipase**.
- They are **lipid soluble molecules** that are **secreted** as they **are formed.**
- Hence they are both **paracrine** and **autocrine signalling molecules** which **activate G-protein-linked receptors** in the **plasma membrane.**
- **Steroid hormones** are **lipid signalling mole-cules** that act mainly by **altering gene trans-cription.**
- As they are **lipids,** they **cannot** be **stored in membrane-bound vesicles** and are therefore **secreted as they are formed.**

c. Signalling in CNS

- In CNS, nerve cells and their connections, bring about signalling.
- The **white matter** contains **large myelinated** nerve **fibers**
- The **grey** matter contains large number of nerve **cell bodies.**
- The **end-feet of** the **astrocytes** form part of the **blood-brain barrier** that **isolates the extra-cellular** fluid around the neurons from changes in **the composition of blood.**
- The **myelin** of axons in **CNS** is formed by **oligo-dendrocytes.**
- **Myelination** of the **peripheral nerve** fibre is done by **Schwann cell**.
- The **axons** of the **peripheral nerves** are protected by **three layers** of connective tissue, i.e. **epineurium, perineurium** and **endoneurium**.
- All **peripheral axons** are **associated** with **Schwann cells** but only the **larger fibres** are covered by **layers of myelin.**
- **Efferent** (motor) **fibres** convey **action potentials** from the **CNS to target** organs, while **afferent (sensory)** fibres convey action potentials from **sense organs** and other **receptors** to **CNS.**
- **Once stimulus intensity** has reached **threshold** level, an **action potential** is **elicited**, but its **amplitude does not increase** further with **increasing stimulus strength.**
- The **action potential** is **'all or none'**. When one potential has passed along an axon, the nerve passes through its **refractory period** and a **second potential cannot occur** until the membrane **regains its excitability**.
- Action potentials cannot **summate**.
- The **action potential** of a **single nerve fibre** is caused by a **large change** in the **permeability** of the **membrane** to **sodium**.
- It is **terminated** when the sodium channels are **inactivated**.

- **Myelin thickness** and **internodal distance increase** with **increasing fibre diameter**. Thus large **myelinated nerve** fibres **conduct faster** than small myelinated or unmyelinated fibres.
- If the **myelin sheath** is lost (demyelination) **saltatory conduction cannot occur** and speed of **conduction falls** dramatically.
- If the **motor nerve conduction velocity** is **50 m/sec,** it will take **10 m/sec** time for action potential to reach a muscle that is **0.5 m** from the **cell body**.
- The actions of **synaptic transmitters** are terminated by **enzymatic destruction**, **uptake** or **diffusion** away from the **synaptic region**.
- **IPSPs hyperpolarize** and make the **post synaptic membrane less excitable.**
- The **release of transmitter** in response to **nerve impulse** occurs by **exocytosis** which is **triggered** by entry of **ca^2** into **nerve terminal.**
- The **motor nerve, together** with **muscle fibres** it **innervates** is called a **motor unit.**
- The **end plate potential** is the **result of an increase in the permeability** of the **junctional membrane** to **Na$^+$ and K$^+$**, leading to **depolarisation.**
- The **neuromuscular junctional receptors** are **nicotinic cholinergic receptors** which can be blocked by **curare.**
- If **acetylcholine estrase** is inhibited, the acetyl choline released by the motor nerve endings is **not destroyed** and **can continue to stimulate** the **nicotinic receptors.**
- **Very prolonged** action of **acetyl choline** leads **ultimately to depolarisation** at the **muscle** and **block of neuromuscular transmission**.
- This is called as blockade by **persistent depolarisation.**

Chapter Three

Blood

a. Composition and Function

- Blood is a heterogenous **fluid** (special connective tissue) circulating in the vessels of the body having many functions including **effective transport** system.
- It consists of (a) **cell mass** (corpuscles) and (b) plasma.
- Cell mass includes RBC, WBC, thrombocytes and occasional **plasma cell.**
- The **plasma** includes **water**, **protein**, **lipids**, **electrolytes**, **mineral**, **sugar** and other **substances** like hormones, excretory products, vitamins, gases and enzymes.
- Cell mass constitutes **45%** (PCV) and plasma **55%.**
- Plasma contains **92% water** and **8% solids**.
- Plasma contains following substances:
  a. Plasma proteins (4–8%), albumin, globulin, fibrinogen.
  b. Electrolytes—Na^+, K^+, Cl^- and HCO_3^-.
  c. Minerals—Iron, Iodine, Copper, Zinc, Manganese, Calcium, Phosphorus, Cobalt.
  d. Metabolic products–Urea, Uric acid, Creatinine, Bilirubin, NH_4, H_2CO_3.
  e. High energy compounds– ATP, GTP, CP.
  f. Hormones.
  g. Gases–CO_2, O_2, N_2.
  h. Nutrients–Glucose, fatty acid, amino acid, vitamins.
  i. Enzymes.
  j. H_2O.

- **Serum** is the **plasma** from which **fibrinogen** and **other proteins** involved in **clotting** are **removed** as a result of clotting (serum is plasma minus clotting factors).
- **Functions** of blood include, **respiratory** (carriage of gases), **nutritive** (transport of nutrients to cells), **excretory** (transport of waste products), **homeostasis** (regulation of body water, pH, electrolyte and BP, regulation of body temperature) and body defence (immune responses).
- Bone marrow **puncture** is done at **sternum** or **iliac crest** to collect bone marrow for **making smear** and identification of cells.
- Bone marrow contains **myeloid** (WBC forming cells) and erythroid (RBC forming cells) series of cells. These cells include RBC and precursors, WBC and precursors, platelets and megakaryocytes, plasma cells, pluripotent and committed stem cells.
- Bone marrow **stem cells** are responsible for the production of not only **blood cells** but also **osteoclasts**, **kupffer cells**, **mast cells**, **dendritic cells** and **Langerhans' cells.**
- Bone marrow **transplant** is useful in **aplastic anaemia** and **leukaemia** patients.

b. Properties of Blood

- In the **ABO blood group system**, two **antigens** (Agglutinogens) may be present separately, together on human red cells or be completely absent, giving rise to four groups; **A, B, AB and O**.
- As per **Landsteiner's law**, if an antigen singly or together with another antigen, is present, corresponding antibody or antibodies are absent in the plasma.
- So person of **blood group A**, has anti-B antibody, **group B** has **anti-A antibody**, AB does not have any antibodies and **group O** has both **anti A and anti B** antibodies in plasma.

- Thus blood cells containing **A antigen** will agglutinate with plasma containing **anti A antibody** and **B antigen** with **anti B antibody.**
- For **successful blood transfusion**, the blood of the donor must be **compatible** what that of **recipient.**
- **Cross matching** is therefore done to establish this **compatibility. RBC of donor** are **matched** with **plasma of recipient** and **vice versa**.
- Since blood **group O** does not contain antigen on RBC membrane it would not react with anti A and anti B or both antibodies of blood group B, A and AB.
- Hence blood **group O** is called as **Universal donor.**
- Since blood **group AB** does not contain any anybody i.e. anti A, B or both it can receive any blood of ABO system. It is called as **universal recipient.**
- **Blood volume** is 7-8% of total body weight and plasma accounts for half of it i.e. about 4%.
- **Plasma** is **95%** water, **5% protein**. Albumin constitutes about 60% of total plasma protein.
- Besides **proteins (colloids)** plasma contains **electrolytes (crystalloids).**
- Plasma has **total osmolarity** of about **290 (roughly 300)** mOsm/L.
- **Colloid osmotic** pressure due to protein is only **28 mmHg.**
- Being **smallest** in **molecular size, albumin** contributes **80-90%** i.e. 25 mmHg of colloid osmotic pressure.
- Of the electrolytes, plasma contains **140mmoles/L Na+**, about **4 mmoles/L of K^+**.
- Hence in a .70 kg (reference man):
  Blood volume is **5 litres.**
  RBC count **4.5×10^{12}** cells/L.
  WBC count **1×10^9** cells/L.
  pH of blood is **7.4.**

- Healthy **red blood** cells **survive** in the circulation for about **120** days before being destroyed by **macrophages** in **RES** of body.
- RBCs are about **7 μm** in **diameter.** They are produced in the **red bone marrow** (Ends of long bones, short flat bones) from erythroblasts.
- The **maturation factors** for **erythropoiesis** are **vitamin B_{12}** and **folic acid.** Their deficiency cause **megaloblastic** or **Macrocytic anaemia.**
- **RBCs** are released into the circulation as immature cells called **reticulocytes.**
- Normally 1% **of RBCs** are **reticulocytes,** but increased reticulocytes **(Reticulocytosis)** would mean **reactive bone marrow.**
- **Haemoglobin** is the **pigment** of RBC. Oxygen combines reversibly with it.
- **One gram** of **Haemoglobin** carries about **1.34 ml of O_2.**
- After leaving the lungs, each deciliter of blood contains about **20 ml of O_2.**
- Each deciliter of **mixed venous blood** contains about 50 ml CO_2.
- **Haemoglobin** is **50% saturated** with O_2 at **PCO_2 of 40 mmHg and PO_2** is about **25 mmHg.**
- **Affinity** of Hb is maximum for **CO** followed by **CO_2** and **O_2**.
- The **platelets** (thrombocytes) count is **250×10^9/L** (2.5 lac ml) i.e. about one platelet for every 20 RBC.
- Platelets are **derived** from **shedding of buds** of **Megakaryocytes** in the bone marrow. These cells are very sticky and adhere to walls of the damaged vessels. Platelets **aggregate** in the presence of **thromboxane A_2**.
- In **dengue fever,** platelet count is very **low** leading to petechial spots all over the body.
- There are **extrinsic** and **intrinsic** pathways for thromboplastin formation and activation of factor X.
- Since intrinsic mechanism involves many factors, it takes longer time as compared to extrinsic.

- Blood clotting depends upon specific clotting factors (about 14 in number) most of them are produced in liver.
- Hemostasis is impaired when platelet count falls below 20×10^9/L. Clotting is initiated by tissue factor coming in contact with blood.
- Primary values of haemogram are:
  Hb: 15G%, RBC count 5 million/mm3.
  PCV : 45%.
  From these other values can be calculated for complete haemogram

$$\text{MCV: } \frac{\text{PCV}}{\text{RBC count}} \times 10 = 90 - 100\,\mu^3$$

$$\text{MCH: } \frac{\text{Hb\%}}{\text{RBC count}} \times 10 = 28 - 32\,\mu\,\text{gm}$$

$$\text{MCHC: } \frac{\text{Hb\%}}{\text{PCV}} \times 100 = 32 - 34\%$$

$$\text{CI: } \frac{\text{Hb as \% of normal}}{\text{RBC count as \% of normal}} \text{ usually } 1$$

- Most of the plasma proteins excluding **γ-globulins** are synthesised in **liver**, hence in liver degenerative disease or cirrhosis of liver plasma protein level decreases causing **hypoproteinemia** and generalized **oedema**.
- Gamma globulins are synthesised by plasma cells and B **lymphocytes**.
- Formation of clots inside blood vessels is called **thrombosis**. They are prone to occur in blood vessels where flow is **sluggish** i.e. in veins of the legs after operation and delivery.
- **Embolism**—bits of thrombus may get separated from parent clot and may get lodged in distant organ causing embolism. Examples are obstruction of pulmonary artery or its branches by thrombi from leg veins (pulmonary embolism).

- **Lymph** is a tissue fluid which enters lymphatic vessels, drains into **venous** blood via the **thoracic** and right lymphatic ducts.
- Lymph contains **proteins**, **clotting factors** **lymphocytes** and the one from intestine is rich in absorbed **fats** and is thus **white** in colour after meals.

c. Hb and RBC

- **Stages** for **erythropoiesis** include, haemocytoblast, burst or colony forming cells, proerythroblast, early, intermediate, late normoblast, reticulocyte and RBC.
- **Reticulocytes** have roughly same size as RBC (8–9 μm) but have **reticulum** due to presence of **remnant RNA.**
- Normal reticulocyte count is **1% of RBC** and **index** is above 2, less than 2 indicates **depressed** bone marrow activity.
- Reticulocyte index

$$= \frac{\text{Reticulocyte count} \times \text{PCV of the patient}}{\text{Normal PCV}}$$

- During the process of erythropoiesis, gross changes in the **maturing cells** include, reduction in **size, loss** of divisibility **disappearance** of RNA, **changes** of basophilic cytoplasm to acidophilic, **appearance** of Hb, **loss** of nucleus and **loss** of mitochondria.
- Normal **life span** of RBC is about **120 days** in circulation but when stored outside, life span is only 3–4 weeks.
- Main functions of RBC are: **transport** of O_2 and CO_2, **acid base** balance. RBC contributes to **viscosity** of blood and influences ESR.
- Various **factors** regulating **erythropoiesis** include; **anoxia** (producing erythropoietin), nutrients (carbohydrate for energy, lipids for membrane and proteins for synthesis of globin, minerals (iron, copper, cobalt and manganese),

maturation factors (vit. B_{12} and folic acid) and **hormones** (thyroid, adrenal cortex, sex hormones growth hormone).

- Physiological **polycythemia** is seen in **new born, high altitude, muscular exercise.**
- Physiological **decrease** in RBC count is seen during **infancy** and **childhood**, **pregnancy** and **old age.**
- **Pathological** conditions giving rise to **polycythemia** include; **polycythemia vera, congenital heart disease, chronic lung disease, leukaemia, cushing syndrome** and **hyperthyroidism.**
- Haemoglobin (Hb) is a **conjugated** protein consisting of **haeme** and **globin.**
- **Haem** is **iron protoporphyrin IX type III** and globin consists of **four polypeptide chains.**
- A single **molecule** of Hb consists of **four protoporphyrin mols** + four **ferrous atoms** + four **polypeptide chains.**
- One **gram** of **Hb** contains about **3.38 mg** of Fe^{++} and has mol weight of **68000**. A normal **adult** Hb contains 2α and 2β **polypeptide chains.**
- There are **five** types of Hb:
  a. Hb A (adult) globin having **2α and 2β** chains.
  b. Hb F (fetal) present in foetus, disappears after birth, globin consists of **2α and 2γ chains**—has more affinity for O_2 at low tensions than Hb A has less affinity to 2, 3 DPG than Hb A.
  c. Hb S (sickle) globin **having 2α and 2β** abnormal chains as **valine** replaces **glutamic** acid in 6th position of β chain. Reduced Hb S causes **sickling** of RBC.
  d. Hb A_2– present in thalassemia patient, globin consists of **2α and 2δ chains.**
  e. Hb C–globin having **2α and 2β** abnormal chains, **glutamic** acid is replaced by **lysine.**
- **Jaundice** is the yellow coloration of skin, conjunctiva and mucus membranes, caused by deposition of excess **bilirubin** in plasma and tissue fluids.

- **Normal** range of bilirubin in health is **0.2–0.8 mg/ 100 ml.**
- Excess plasma bilibrubin may be due to:
  a. Excessive RBC **break down** (haemolytic or prehepatic jaundice).
  b. **Infective** or **toxic damage** of liver cells (hepatic jaundice).
  c. **Obstruction** of bile ducts (obstructive jaundice).
- **Anaemia** is defined as a **quantitative** or **qualitative reduction** in RBC count leading to a **decreased O_2 carrying** capacity. Usually RBC count and Hb levels are low.
- Basis of classification of anaemia:
  a. Due to **decreased** production of RBC.
  b. Due to **excessive loss** of blood.
  c. Due to **increased destruction** of RBC.

d. Anaemia

- Anaemia due to **decreased production** of RBC could be due to:
  a. **Nutritional deficiency** (raw materials to factory are deficient)—this includes **megaloblastic** anaemia (deficiency of vit B_{12} and folic acid) **microcytic hypochromic** anaemia (deficiency of iron).
  b. **Hypoplastic** bone marrow (factory is not working properly despite getting all raw materials) hypo activity of bone marrow may be due to **damage** caused by **drugs, toxins, radiations.**
  c. **Renal** and **thyroid** disease (lack of erythropoietin or T_3, T_4) adversely affects erythropoieses.
- Anaemia due to **excess loss** of blood: It could be due to acute haemorrhage, accidental or menorrhagia (excessive menstrual bleeding) piles or hook worm infestation–normochromic, normocytic anaemia develops.

- **Anaemia** due to **increased destruction** of RBC–called as **haemolytic anaemias,** due to corpuscular (spherocytosis, sickle cell, thalassemia, G6PD deficiency, methaemoglobinemias) or **extra corpuscular** defects (antibodies against RBC, drugs, snake venom, hypersplenism).
- ESR (BSR) is also referred to as suspension stability of blood expressed as settling down of RBC under influence of gravity as mm/hr.
- Normal ESR by **wintrobe's** method in male is: 0-9 mm/hr, female: 0-20 mm/hr.
  Westergen method, male: 0-5 mm/hr, female: 0-7 mm/hr.
- ESR depends on rouleaux formation (piling up of RBC) which is assisted by fibrinogen.
- ESR is raised in pathological states like, tuberculosis, malignancy, pyogenic infections, rheumatic fever, rheumatoid arthritis and nephrosis.
- ESR differentiates between organic or functional disorders, raised in the former.

e. WBC and Platelets

- **Physiological** leucocytosis (count> 12000/mm^3) is seen in muscular **exercise, after meals, emotions, high altitude** and in **newborn and infants.**
- **Pathological** states showing leucocytosis include, **fever** (except typhoid and viral) **leukaemias, myocardial infarction, pyogenic infections.**
- Leucopenia (WBC < 4000/ mm^3) is seen in pathological states like, **aplastic anaemia, viral infection, typhoid.**
- **Neutrophilia** is commonly seen in, **pyogenic infections, myocardial infarction, malignant neoplasm** and **acute inflammation** like appendicitis, pneumonia.
- **Eosinophilia** (rise in eosinophil count) is seen in **asthma, parasitic infestations, hay fever, allergies** and **tropical** eosinophilia.

- Important functions of **spleen** are: its RES participates in **storage** of **iron**, **destruction** of **senile RBC** and **Hb**, **phagocytose** foreign organism and **participate** in development of **immunity.** Spleen also **stores** RBCs, produces **lymphocytes** and has **haemopoeitic** function during **fetal life.**
- **Primary** functions of **plasma proteins** are: maintenance of **colloid osmotic** pressure (mainly albumin), **viscosity** of blood (directly related to peripheral resistance), **regulate acid base** balance (act as buffers), act as **protein reserve** (used during starvation), **influence ESR** (fibrinogen), **transport** of CO_2, hormones and minerals (transferrin, ceruloplasmin, TBG and CBG).
- Hypoproteinaemia refers to **low plasma** protein level (normal being 4.5 to 7.5 gm%) and causes **oedema** (accumulation of fluid in interstitial spaces).
- The common causes of **hypoproteinaemia** and thus oedema are; **cirrhosis** of liver (liver not working), **nephrotic** syndrome (albuminuria), **malnutrition** (less raw material), **starvation** and **malabsorption** syndrome.
- **Platelets** play important role in **clotting** as they contain several clotting factors, phospholipids and thrombosthenin. All these help in **clot formation** and **retraction.** Platelet factor 3 converts prothrombin to thrombin.
- The **intrinsic** activators of plasminogen to plasmin, include factor XIIa, kallikrein, factor XIa and activated protein C.
- The **extrinsic** activators are; vascular plasminogen activator from endothelium, urokinase (kidney), streptokinase (from streptococcus) and trypsin.
- **Anti coagulants** commonly used in **laboratory** include, K^+, NH^4 **double oxalate** (precipitates Ca^{++}), **Na^+ citrate 3.8%** (forms double salt with Ca^{++}), **Na_2SO_4** (forms compound with Ca^{++}),

EDTA (precipitates Ca^{++}) and **Na^+ fluoride** (weak compound formed with Ca^{++}).

- Common **tests** used for evaluating **bleeding,** clotting disorders are; clotting and bleeding time **(BTCT), prothrombia time, thromboplastin generation test, Hess capillary** fragility test, **platelet count** and **clot retraction time.**
- Whole blood **transfusion** is indicated in patients of **severe bleeding** or bleeding during operation.
- Blood **substitutes** like (packed RBC, platelet concentrate, WBC concentrate, plasma, saline, albumin and clotting factor concentrate) are transfused in **mild haemorrhage, dehydration, burns** and **bleeding disorders**.
- **Immediate** effects of **mismatched** blood transfusion include, **chills** and **rigors, fever** and **headache, breathlessness, joint pains, chest** and **abdominal pain, nausea** and **vomiting** and **patient can go into shock.**

f. Haemostasis

- The initial response to blood vessel injury is vasoconstriction, as well as sticking together of the opposed endothelial surfaces.
- The next events are formation of platelet plug followed by blood clotting.
- 'Capillary fragility test' is used to assess capillary resistance to injurious influences.
- Platelets adhere to the exposed collagen in a damaged vessel and release the content of their secreting vesicles, which further enhance platelet aggregation.
- This process is also enhanced by Von willebrand factor, secreted by the endothelium and by thrombosane A_2, produced by platelets.

g. Blood Clot Formation

- Blood is transformed into **solid gel**, when at site of damage, plasma **fibrinogen** is converted into **fibrin** molecules, which form a **meshwork.**

- This reaction is catalyzed by **enzyme thrombin,** which also activates **factor XIII,** a plasma protein which **stabilises** fibrin.
- The formation thrombin from the plasma protein **prothrombin** is the **end** result of **cascade** of **reactions** in which an **inactive** plasma **protein** is activated and then **enzymatically** activates the next **protein** in the **series.**
- In the **intrinsic** pathways, the cascade begins with activation of **factor XII,** by contact with collagen underlying damaged vessels.
- In the **extrinsic** clotting pathway, the cascade begins when tissue factor forms an active complex with plasma **factor VII,** and this complex activates factor IX and X, plugging into intrinsic pathway at this point.
- Both **Ca^{++}** and **platelet phospholipid** are required at **several steps** in the **cascade.**
- Two of the factors involved in clotting, factor VIII and V are activated in a **positive feedback** manner by **thrombin.**
- Vitamin **K** is required by the **liver** for normal production of some of the **clotting factors.**
- Clotting time **increases** in **deficiency** of clotting factors like deficiency of **factor VIII** causing haemophilia.

h. Anticlotting Systems

- Clotting is opposed by protein C and antithrombin III.
- Protein C is activated by thrombin and inactivates factors VIII, V.
- Antithrombin III binds, to heparin on endothelial cells and inactivates thrombin.
- Clots are dissolved by the fibrinolytic system in which the plasma pre-enzyme, plasminogen, is activated by plasminogen activator to plasmin, which digests fibrin.
- Tissue plasminogen activator is secreted by endothelial cells and is activated by fibrin in a clot.

- Plasmins (fibrinolysin) dissolve the intravascular clots.

i. Inflammation and Immunity

- Tissue **transplantation** from one person to another to treat **organ failure** has been a major goal of medicine. The first such procedure was the **transfusion** of blood after proper direct and cross matching.
- Successful skin **grafts** or organ **transplant** require a **close** match between the **specific cell markers** of both **donor** and **recipient**.
- Individuals having **similar genetic** make up like **monovular** twins (identical twins) and tissue antigens (MHC or in human HLA) can receive or donate organs successfully.
- The tissue **graft rejection** is an **immunological** phenomenon and paved the way for successful skin and organ transplants between individuals of different **genetic** background.
- The solution of graft rejection is to (a) match the tissue of the donor as closely as possible with that of the recipients (tissue typing) and (b) to inhibit the activity of the immune system with **immuno-suppressant** drugs.
- This approach has proved very successful with **skin grafts**, **kidney** and **heart** transplants with 5 years or more survival rate of 70-80%.
- Close tissue matching is not needed for **corneal grafts** because the cornea does not become **vascularized** and so is not subject to attacks by the lymphocytes.
- Grafts of the skin from healthy part of the body to injured part of an individual is called as **autograft** and grafting skin from some one else is known as **allografts.**
- There are two primary immune responses (a) **Humoral** antibody formation (b) **cell mediated** immune response.

- **B** lymphocytes mediate the first one and **T lymphocytes** second one.
- Antibodies (Immunoglobulins) **bind** with the antigen to **neutralize** its effect. Whereas T lymphocytes attack the virulent organism/foreign cells to **destroy** them.
- There are **five** types of **immunoglobulins** i.e. IgG, IgA, IgM, IgD IgE.
- Neutrophils pass from the circulation into the tissues in response to chemotactic stimuli (**Chemotaxis**). They phagocyte and kill invading micro-organisms.
- Macrophages use nitric oxide (NO) (and reactive oxygen intermediates) to kill organisms they have ingested.
- The **monocytes** of the blood are the precursors of tissue **macrophages**.
- Complement facilitates uptake of bacteria by phagocytes.
- Natural **killer cells** act by destroying cells infected with **virus**.
- The first stage of the inflammatory response is vasodilatation (the red reaction of the triple response).
- The capillaries at the site of inflammation become highly **permeable** and exude plasma.
- **Mast cells** secrete chemotactic and vasoactive substances (**prostaglandins** and **leukotriens**) during inflammation.
- The neutrophils are the most abundant of the WBCs (about 70% in adults) followed by lymphocytes which accounts for 25% WBCs of the blood.
- **Lymphocytes** leave the circulation to migrate through the tissues, finally re-entering the blood via the **thoracic duct.**
- B lymphocytes are processed in the bone marrow or Bursa Fabricius and some of them are transformed into plasma cells and secrete antibody, others remain in lymphoid tissue as memory cells.

- T lymphocytes are derived from stem cells in the bone marrow and mature in the **thymus** gland (hence name T lymphocytes).
- Only the **cytotoxic** T cells secrete cytotoxic material to kill target cell.
- **Helper** T cells secrete **cytokines**.
- T cells respond to MHC molecules of foreign cell and proteins on the host cells.
- **IgM** being **larger** molecule does not **cross placenta** whereas **IgG** can cross it and protects the foetus and neonates from infection.

j. Cells and Chemicals Mediators of Immune Functions

- **Macrophages:** Cells processing antigens and presenting antigens to lymphocytes.
- **B cells:** Immunocompetent **lymphocytes**, which upon activation, proliferate and differentiate into **antibody** secreting **plasma cells,** provide major defence against bacteria, virus in extra cellular fluid and toxins. Can also function as antigen processing cells for helper T cells.
- **Cytotoxic T cells:** Class of **T lymphocytes,** that on activation by specific antigen, directly attack the cells bearing that type of antigen; with NK cells and effector macrophages, are major killers of virus infected cells and tumor cells.
- **Effector macrophages:** Macrophages whose killing ability has been enhanced by **lymphokines,** particularly **gamma interferon.**
- **Eosinophils:** Granulocytes involved in **allergic responses** and destruction of **parasites**.
- **Lymphocytes:** The type of leukocytes responsible for **specific** immune defenses, categorised mainly as **B cells** and **T cells** (NK cells constitute another category).
- **Mast cells:** Cell types derived from **basophils,** release inflammatory mediators in immediate allergy.

- **Monocyte:** A type of leucocyte, leaves the blood steam and is transformed into a **macrophage,** has functions similar to those of macrophages.
- **Memory cells:** B cells that differentiate during an initial infection and respond rapidly during a **subsequent exposure** to the same antigen.
- **Neutrophils:** Granulocytes that function as **phagocytes** and also release chemical involved in inflammation.
- **Plasma cells:** Cells that differentiate from activated **B lymphocytes** and **secrete antibodies** (Immunoglobulins).
- **T cells:** Lymphocytes derived from precursors that differentiate in thymus: categories are cytotoxic, helper and suppressor T cells.
- **Antibodies:** immunoglobulins that function as antigen receptor on **B cells** and secreted by plasma cells, secreted antibodies combine with the antigen that stimulates it and direct an attack against the antigen on cell bearing it.
- **Complement:** A group of plasma **proteins**, that upon activation, kill microbes directly and facilitate the various steps of the inflammatory process including phagocytosis.
- **Cytokines:** Are protein messengers secreted either by macrophages and monocytes or by lymphocytes (lymphokines).
- **Immunoglobulin (Ig):** Synonym for antibody, five major classes are:
  a. *IgA:* Secreted by the lining of the body's various tracts.
  b. *IgD:* Function is unknown.
  c. *IgE:* Mediate immediate hypersensitivity (allergy) and resistance to parasites.
  d. *IgG:* most abundant class of antibody.
  e. *IgM:* along with IgG provide the bulk of specific humoral antibody formation against bacteria and viruses.

- **Interferon:** Class of proteins that non specifically **inhibit** viral replication in addition, gamma interferon stimulates the killing ability of cytotoxic T cells, NK cells and macrophages.
- **Interleukins (IL2):** Proteins secreted by macrophages and (other cells) that causes helper T cells exert many inflammatory effects, and mediates acute phase response.
- **Interleukin (IL-1):** Protein secreted by macrophages and (other cells) that cause helper T cells exert many inflammatory effects, and mediate acute phase response.
- **Interleukin 2 (IL-2):** Protein secreted by activated helper T cells that cause helper T cells, cytotoxic T cells, and NK cells to proliferate.
- **Interleukin 6 (IL-6):** Protein secreted by **macrophages** (and other cells) that mediate many of the acute phase response.
- **Membrane attack complex (MAC):** Group of complement protein that forms channels on the surface of microbes making it **leaky** and **killing** it.
- **Platelet activating factor:** Mediator synthesised and released by mast cells that stimulates inflammation.
- **Tumor necrosis factor:** Monokines that kill target cells out right, stimulate inflammation and many of the system acute phase responses.
- **Prostaglandins:** Class of cricosenoids that function as inflammation mediators.

Chapter Four

Cardiovascular System

a. General Features

- In a normal subject, most of the blood **volume** is **located** in the systemic **veins** (capacitance vessels).
- The **colloid** osmotic pressure of blood is mainly determined by the plasma concentration of **albumin.**
- **Neural** regulation of **vascular resistance** in skeletal muscles depends on the activity of the **sympathetic nerves** to muscle.
- During the so-called **resting** membrane potential of myocardial cell, the transmembrane potential depends on **conductance** of **potassium.**
- A–V nodal fibres of the heart junctional tissue display property of post repolarisation **refractoriness.**
- In a typical systemic capillary, the tension in its wall increases as the **hydrostatic pressure** rises.
- The **mean** arterial pressure in **pulmonary** circulation is much **lower** than systemic because resistance to blood flow is **lower** in **pulmonary** circuit as compared to systemic.
- Velocity of shortening of myocardial fibres is **greatest** when **preload** is moderate and after load is **zero.**
- The capillary fluid **exchange** into interstitial spaces **increases** as the tissue hydrostatic pressure **decreases.**

- The most important cause of **increase** in blood flow in **exercising muscles** is due to vasodilatory action of **local** metabolites.
- An increase in ventricular contractility is indicated by increase in **stroke volume** and decrease in **end diastolic volume.**
- **Most** effective stimulation for medullary vasomotor centre is the **increase** in **arterial PCO_2.**
- **Stroke volume** is always **greater** in a physically **trained** (athelete) person than **untrained** one.
- A reduction in mean arterial pressure results in a reflex which increases **total peripheral** resistance.
- The highly vascular organ (blood flow/gm/min) in the body is carotid bodies.
- A sudden hypovolemic shock (acute haemorrhage) causes decrease in stroke volume and decrease in central venous pressure.
- Velocity of blood flow is **maximum** in **aorta.**
- **Severe** exercise results in an increase in **arteriovenous** oxygen **difference.**
- **Metabolic** activity of **myocardium** mostly regulates the **coronary blood flow.**
- Cardiac contractility is enhanced by administration of beta blockers.
- The two principle determinants of **mean arterial** pressure are: **cardiac output** and **peripheral resistance.**
- First response to sudden exposure to high attitude hypoxia is increase in respiration.

b. Heart

- The **ejection** fraction of the heart is ratio between **stroke volume** and **end diastolic volume.**
- In the coronary circulation, **extraction** of **oxygen** by **myocardium** is high, hence venous O_2 content is one of the **lowest** in the body.
- In an organ metabolically active, **blood flow** and **tissue metabolism** are **directly** related.

- The **rate** of conduction velocity is higher in **purkinje** fibres as compared to **atria** or **ventricles.**
- During **isometric** relaxation phase of cardiac cycle, **all valves** are **closed.**
- The **action potential** of **skeletal muscle** is about **2 ms** in duration, while that of the **heart cells** range from **150 ms** in the cells of **SA node** to about 300 ms in the **Purkinje fibre**.
- Hence on an **average action potentials** in the heart are about **100 times** longer than those of **skeletal muscle.**
- The **membrane potential** of the **SA node** (pacemaker) cells is low, **about - 60 mV**, while that of **ventricular cells** is **about -90 mV.**
- Although the **conduction** of the **cardiac impulse** through the **atria** occurs **preferentially** via certain **fibre bundles,** these cells are, nevertheless, normal **atrial myocytes.**
- The **transmission** of **cardiac** impulses in the ventricle is through bundle cells and the purkinje fibres which transmit their **action potentials** to **myocytes** via **gap junctions**.
- The **P wave** of **ECG** reflects **atrial depolarization** and **proceeds atrial contraction**.
- The **QRS complex** reflects the **time** during which **ventricular** fibres **are depolarised.**
- The **T wave** reflects the **repolarization** of the **ventricular** fibres.
- The **P-Q interval** is normally about **0.1 sec.**
- The **peak amplitude** of the ECG is about **1 mV.**
- The **volume** of blood in the **ventricles** at the end of **diastole (end diastolic volume)** is about **120 ml**.
- Of this about **70 ml** is ejected **(stroke volume)** and rest 50 ml remains in **ventricles (end systolic volume).**
- The **ratio** of the **stroke volume** to the end-diastolic **volume** is called the **ejection fraction** and is usually about **60%** at **rest.**

- During **ventricular diastole** the **pressure** in **left ventricle** is close to **zero.**
- During **ventricular systole** the **pressure** in **left ventricle** reaches a **maximum** of about 16 kPa **(120 mmHg).**
- During the **first phase of ventricular systole,** the **volume** of the ventricle **does not change.**
- **The** first heart sound corresponds with the **closure of the mitral** and **tricuspid valves.**
- First heart sound **occurs** after the **onset of ventricular contraction,** which **follows the R wave.** Approximately it marks the **beginning of systole.**
- The **second heart** sound is caused by **closure** of the **aortic** and **pulmonary valves.**
- This **occurs** at the **end of ventricular systole,** when the ventricles have **repolarized.** So it marks the **end of systole** or **beginning of diastole.**
- Hence **time period** between **first** and **second** heart sound **corresponds** to **ventricular systole** and between second and **first heart** sound marks the **ventricular diastole.**
- So **first heart** sound follows **R wave** and **second follows T wave** of **ECG.**
- About the **cardiac output:**
  a. It is the **volume** of blood **pumped out** by **each ventricle per minute**—about 5L.
  b. It is **a product** of **stroke volume** × **heart rate** (SV is 70 ml × 72 min about 5L/min).
  c. The cardiac output is, **on average,** the **same** for **both left** and **right sides** of the **heart.**
  d. The cardiac output is **measured** by **dividing the O_2 consumption** by the **difference in O_2 content** between **mixed venous** and **arterial blood.**
  e. Cardiac output can be **increased** by **circulating catecholamines.**
- **Arterial blood pressure depends** on **cardiac output** and **total peripheral resistance.**

- **Mean arterial BP** is given by the **sum of** the **diastolic pressure** and **one-third** of the **pulse pressure.**
- **Pulse pressure** is **difference** between **systolic** and **diastolic pressure**.
- The **main site** of **peripheral resistance** is the **arterioles.**
- The **arterial blood pressure** is normally **16/10.6 kPa** i.e. **120/80 mmHg.**
- The **flow of blood** in the **large veins** is **pulsatile.**
- The **peripheral resistance depends** on **state of the arterioles.**
- The **arterioles** are **under nervous, hormonal** and **local control**.
- **Autoregulation** of **flow occurs** in **denervated blood vessels** and is **an intrinsic property—two mechanism** appear to be involved (a) local metabolites and (b) **myogenic response** of the smooth muscle **to stretch.**
- **Reactive hyperaemia** is due to **vasodilatation** caused by accumulation of metabolites during a period of occluded blood flow.
- **Activation** of the **sympathetic** system causes vasoconstriction in the **viscera** and **skin** but **vasodilation** in **skeletal muscles**.
- **Parasympathetic vasodilator** fibres innervate the **blood vessels of GIT.**
- The **process of exchange** between **capillaries** and **tissues** occurs mainly **through diffusion.**
- The **plasma proteins** (through their colloid osmotic pressure) play an **important role** in tissue **fluid exchange**.
- A **fraction** of the **fluid** that leaves the **capillaries** at the **arteriolar end** is **reabsorbed** by the **capillaries** at the venous end and by **pericytic venules**.
- The **fraction that** is **not absorbed** is **returned** to the circulation via **the lymph**.
- The **lymph** has **same ionic composition** as the plasma but has a **lower oncotic** pressure.

- On **sudden fall** in **arterial blood pressure** (acute **haemorrhage)** the **baroreceptor** are less active and this **increases sympathetic activity** in the cardiac and **vasoconstrictor nerves.**
- Hence **heart rate** and **peripheral vascular resistance increase restoring** blood pressure to **normal**.
- The **coronary blood flow** is **mainly regulated** by **metabolic hyperemia**.
- The **cardiac volume receptor** are **mainly responsible** for the **long-term regulation** of systemic **blood pressure**.

c. Integration of CVS Functions

- **Veins** serve as **low resistant condicts** for **venous return**.
- Veins are very **compliant** and contain most of the blood in the vascular system. Hence they serve as **capacitance** vessels.
- **Diameter** of veins is **reflexly** altered by **vaso-constriction/vasodilation** so as to maintain **venous pressure** and venous return.
- The skeletal **muscle pump** and **respiratory muscle** pump increase venous **pressure locally** and enhance **venous return** to the **heart** (venous valves make flow one sided towards heart).
- **Mean arterial pressure**, the primary regulated variable in CVS, **equals** the **product** of **cardiac output** and total **peripheral resistance**.
- The **primary baroceptors** are the **arterial baroreceptors** located in two **carotid sinusess** and the **aortic arch** innervated by sinus nerve (branch of glossopharyngeal) and aortic nerve (branch of vagus).
- **Non arterial** baroreceptors are located in the systemic **veins, pulmonary vessels** and walls of **heart**.
- The **firing rates** of the arterial **baroreceptors** are **proportional** to **mean arterial pressure** and **pulse pressure**.

- An **increase** in arterial baroreceptor **firing** due to increase in pressure through **medullary CVS centres** causes an **increase** in **parasympathetic outflow** and **decrease** in sympathetic **outflow** to the **heart, arterioles and veins**—resulting in **decrease** in **cardiac output** and **total peripheral resistance** and hence **decrease** in **mean arterial pressure**.
- The **opposite** occurs i.e. rise in mean arterial pressure, when the **initial** change is a **decrease** in **arterial pressure (hypotension/shock).**
- The **baroreceptor reflexes** (sinuarotic mechanism) are short term **regulatory** mechanics for BP, but **adapt** to a **maintained** change in BP.
- The most **important long term** regulation of mean arterial pressure is the **blood volume**.
- **Shock** is any situation in which blood flow to tissues/organs is **low** enough to cause damage.
- In the **upright posture**, pooling of blood occurs in **veins** and **capillaries** of **limbs** due to pull of **gravity** on unbroken **vascular columns**.
- The **increased** venous pressure distends. The veins, and the increased capillary pressure increases **filtration** out of capillaries.
- Therefore prolonged **standing** in attention can cause, low **venous return**, **low cardiac output** and BP **(postural hypotension)** and thereby **decreased** blood flow to **brain** causing **syncope**.
- Hence such **professionals** (Police, army personnel) are advised to **contract** their **skeletal muscles** in the leg quite **often** to minimise pooling of blood.
- **Distribution** of **cardiac output** to different organs per min at rest is: **brain** 750 ml, **Heart** 250 ml, **Muscles** 1200 ml, **Skin** 500 ml, **Kidney** 1100 ml, **Abdominal organs** 1400 ml and **others** 600 ml, total **being 5800 ml/min (cardiac output)**.
- During **strenuous exercise**, cardiac output **increases three fold** and blood flows/min is : brain **750 ml**, heart **750 ml**, muscles **12500 ml**,

Skin **1900 ml**, Kidney **600 ml**, abdominal organs **600 ml**, others **400 ml**.

- Thus there is **tremendous increase** in **muscle** blood flow, moderate increase in coronary and **skin blood** flow. Whereas flow to kidney and abdominal **organs** (splanchnic) is **reduced** during exercise.
- The **changes** in **CVS** during **exercise** are due to **active hyperaemia** in the **skeletal muscle** and **heart**, increased **sympathetic output** to the **heart** (positive inotropic and chronotropic effect), **arterioles** and **veins** and **decreased parasympathetic** outflow to heart.
- The **increase** in cardiac **output**, besides sympathetic stimulation to heart is also due to **factors** helping increase in **venous return**.
- **Training** can **increase** person's **stroke volume** and thus **maximum** indurance.

d. Regional Circulation

- **Specific regulatory mechanism** are used in **localised** regions of the **cardiovascular system** to **match** flow to **tissue requirements**.
- The **coronary circulation** has to provide the **myocardium** with **sufficient blood** to meet its metabolic demands despite the **compression** of coronary vessels that occurs during each **contraction**.
- Hence **coronay blood** flow is regulated largely by local mutabilities, including **adenosine, CO_2, H^+**, and **K^+.** there is a **close parallel between metabolic activity** and **blood flow**.
- The **principal role** of **cutaneous circulation** is in **thermoregulation**, achieved through **large variation** in **blood flow. Specialised vessels,** the **arteriovenous anastomosis constrict** in **response to sympathetic nerve activity** to **shunt** blood from the **arterioles directly** to **the venules.** This **occurs** as a **mechanism** to **conserve body heat (Exposure to cold).**

- **Blood flow** to **skeletal muscle varies** directly with their activity. During exercise, **vasodilatation occurs** in response to local **build up of metabolities—functional hyperaemia**.
- **Sustained muscle** contraction may **compress the vessels, occluding them, metabolities** then **accumulate quickly** and cause **reactive hyperaemia** and the **circulation** is **restored.**
- **Brain tissue** has **high capillary** density, cerebral blood is **kept within narrow limits** by **autoregulation, local metabolic control** and **reflexes initiated by brain** itself.. **Hypercapnia** causes **vasodilatation,** mediated by **nitric oxide**.
- All of the **output** of the **right ventricle** passes through the **pulmonary circulation** and the output of both ventricles will be the same.
- The **systolic** and **diastolic pressure** in pulmonary circulation are about 25 and 8 mmHg respectively as compared to 120/80 mmHg for **systemic arteries**.
- Although the pressure in the **pulmonary arteries rise** with **increasing cardiac output,** the increase is **small as the resistance of the pulmonary** circulation **falls.**
- While the **lungs inactivate many vasoactive** materials i.e., **bradykinin,** they convert **angiotensin I** to **angiotensin II**.
- In an **upright individual,** pulmonary **blood flow** is **greatest** at the **base of the lung.**
- The **pattern of pulmonary** blood flow is dependent on posture.

e. CVS Pattern in Disease

- **Hypertension** (raised BP) is usually due to **increased** total **peripheral resistance** resulting from increased **arteriolar constriction**.
- More than **95%** of hypertension is termed as **primary** (Essential) as cause of increased arteriolar constriction is **not known**.

- Systolic > **140** and diastolic > **90** mmHg recorded at **three** different days, is labelled as **raised BP**.
- **Heart failure** is a decreased cardiac **contractility** such that cardiac output is **inadequate**.
- It leads to **fluid retention** by the **kidneys** and formation of **oedema** because of increased **capillary pressure**.
- Pulmonary **oedema** can occur when left ventricle **fails**.
- **Insufficient** coronary **blood flow** can cause **damage** to the **heart**.
- **Acute death** from a **heart attack** is usually due to **ventricular fibrillation**.
- The major **cause** of **reduced** coronary blood **flow** is **atherosclerosis**, an **occlusive** disease of the **arteries**.
- Persons may suffer from **intermittent** attacks of **angina pectoris** without actually suffering a heart attack at the time of pain.
- **Atherosclerosis** can also cause **cerebral strokes**, and symptoms of inadequate **blood flow** (ischaemia) in other **areas** (Peripheral vascular disease, causing ischaemic pain in the limbs).
- Vascular **endothelium** plays important role in maintaining patency of blood vessels, blood flow and arterial pressure—**Vascular homeostasis.**
- **Endothelium derived vasoactive factors** (both dilators and constrictors like nitric oxide, endothelin) play important role in **maintaining orderly** and **effective** blood flow in vessels and **blood pressure.**

Chapter Five

Respiration

a. Mechanics of Respiration

- The **trachea** and **bronchi** have cartilaginous rings that allow them to **stay open** despite changes in **intrapleural pressure.**
- Since the **bronchioles lack** this cartilage, they **collapse** when the **intrapulmonary pressure** exceeds the **pressure in the airway.**
- The principal sites of **airway resistance** are the upper airways. The fall in resistance with the **branching of airways** is the result of a very **large increase** in **total cross sectional area**.
- While the **alveoli** are the **main sites** of **gas exchange**, the **respiratory bronchioles** and **alveolar ducts** also **take part** in gas exchange.
- In a **healthy lung** the **distance** between the **alveolar** air and **the blood in the pulmonary capillaries** is less than **1 µm.**
- In a **normal healthy** man:
  a. **Total lung capacity** is about 6L.
  b. **The tidal volume** at rest is about **500 ml**.
  c. The **vital capacity** is equal to total lung volume minus residual volume. i.e. 6-1 = 5L.
  d. **Functional residual capacity** (FRC) is equal to ERV + RV e.g. 1+1 = **2 litres**.
  e. FEV_1 (forced expiratory volume first sec). would be 3/5 L i.e. 70% of vital capacity.
- The **compliance** of the chest **(Thorax)** is determined by that of the **chest wall and the lungs.**

- **Lung recoil assists expiration,** but not **inspiration** which is an active process.
- **Pulmonary surfactant reduces** the **work of breathing** by lowering the **surface tension** of the **air-liquid interface** in **alveoli.**
- The **surface tension** is **related** to the **degree of inflation:** The **more** the lungs are **expanded**, the **higher the surface tension**.
- **Compliance** is defined as **change in volume** of lungs with **change in pressure.**
- The **compliance** of the lungs is **determined by surface tension forces** in the **alveoli** and by the **elastic tissues** of the **lung parenchyma**.
- At the **functional residual volume,** the **elastic recoil** of the **lungs** is **balanced** by the **elastic forces, tending to expand the chest.**
- The **physiological dead space** is always **greater** than the **anatomical** dead space as it **includes the volume** of **air taken** up by **alveoli** that are not **perfused** by blood and therefore **cannot** take part in **gas exchange.**
- When **lungs are expanded** during inspiration, **dead space increases** with **increase** in **tidal volume.**
- **Alveolar ventilation** is **greatest** at the **base of the lungs** for **lung volume at** or **above FRC**.
- For lung volume less than FRC, the ventilation at apex is greater than that at the base.
- While the **volumes** of **CO_2 and O_2 exchanged** during respiration are **similar,** the **pressure gradients** for **CO_2** is **much smaller**.
- This is **offset** by the much **greater diffusing** capacity of **CO_2 (about 20 times** that of **O_2).**
- **The** V_A/Q_A ratio for a **subject** in a **sitting position increases** with distance above **base** of the lungs.
- The **regional variation** in V_AQ_A ratio is **much smaller** in subjects who are **lying down.**
- The **respiratory muscles** are **striated skeletal muscles** and have **no intrinsic/spontaneous**

rhythm. Their **rhythmical** activity is **derived** from the activity of **their motoneurons.**

- The **basic neural machinery** for **generation** of the **respiratory rhythm** is located in the **lower medulla.**
- Hence **respiration** will **continue** even if **all afferents** are **cut**.
- The **main muscle** of respiration is **diaphragm.**
- **During expiration** the activity of the **external intercostal** muscles is **inhibited** (as expiration is **passive process).**
- The **peripheral chemoreceptors** are the **carotid** and **aortic bodies**, which sense **plasma pH, PO_2 and PCO_2.**
- The **peripheral chemoreceptors** sense **PO_2** and **central chemoreceptors sense PCO_2** in **arterial blood**.
- **Rate and depth** of **breathing increases** on breathing **air with 5% CO_2.**

b. Respiratory Functions

- The **principal function** of lungs is to insure that inspired air and pulmonary blood flow are distributed **adequately** to all lung units so that gas exchange occurs with minimal energy used.
- **Increase** in mean **arterial** or **pulse pressure** stimulates carotid and aortic **baroreceptors** to cause **decrease** in **heart rate**, fall in blood pressure and decrease in respiratory rate.
- Since this **sinu-aortic mechanism** controls **heart rate/BP** under check, it is also referred to as CVS **buffer mechanism** or baroreceptor buffer reflex.
- **Decrease** of PO_2 to about **60 mmHg**, is **a potent** stimulus for **peripheral chemoreceptors** of carotid and aortic bodies.
- Peripheral chemoreceptor stimulation results in hyperpnoea, tachycardia and rise in BP.
- Peripheral chemoreceptors become **insensitive** and non responsive to fall of arterial PO_2 below **30 mmHg**.

- There is relationship between **respiration** and **blood pressure**, during **inspiration** (latter part) heart rate and **BP rises**, this is also the reason for sinus arrhythmia.
- Respiratory **excursion** on **BP recordings** in animals is marked by appearance of waves on BP records called as **Traube Herring waves**.
- The peripheral chemoreceptors are **stimulated** by decrease in **PO_2, increase in PCO_2, decrease in pH** and certain chemicals like **diguniides, Ach**.
- There is **adrenergic efferent** innervation of **peripheral chemoreceptors** which on stimulation enhances chemoreceptor discharge and thus respiration.
- One of the reasons for increase in ventilation during exercise is adrenergic stimulation of peripheral chemoreceptors.
- Herring-Breuer inflation reflex protects lungs from excessive inflation.
- During embryonic period, the lungs first appear at about **24th** day after fertilisation.
- The lungs are mature enough to support life by **24th** week of gestation.
- Number of lung alveoli go on increasing till the age of 12 years.
- The average PO_2 in the umbilical arteries, during fetal life, is 20 mmHg and that in umbilical vein is 40 mmHg.
- The average PCO_2 in the umbilical arteries during fetal life is about 55 mmHg.
- In the fetal circulation, most of the blood entering right atrium passes to the left atrium through foramen ovale.
- Shortly after birth, the ductus arteriosus constricts in response to increased PO_2.
- With advancing age, **vital capacity** and PEFR go on **decreasing.**
- Between 20-25 years of age, most of the **lung indices** reach their maximum level.

- Over the course of life, **diffusion capacity** of the lungs **decreases** by 20%.
- The act of **normal inspiration** is **limited** by inputs coming from **stretch receptors** in lungs, chest wall and peripheral chemoreceptors.
- **Oxidative** energy requirements of the cells determines the normal **basal oxygen** consumption which is usually **200 ml/min**.
- **Alveolar PO_2** regulates **local perfusion** of ventilating units.
- During exercise, **number** of capillaries being perfused in muscles, **increases** which results in **three-fold** increase in **diffusing capacity**.
- **Intrapleural** (intrathoracic) pressure is the pressure that can be recorded from the **intrapleural space**. Its normal value varies with respiration.
- During **inspiration** i/p pressure is **–6 mmHg**, during **forceful inspiration** goes upto **–30 mmHg** and at the **end of expiration** it is **–2.5 mmHg**.
- **Pulmonary function tests** consist of battery of tests which evaluate **ventilation, diffusion** and control of **breathing**.
- **Ventilatory lung function tests** include (a) **static tests** e.g. lung volumes and capacities (spirometry and helium dilution for FRC), pulmonary compliance and maximum expiratory pressure. (b) **Dynamic tests** include, maximum voluntary ventilation (MVV), forced expiratory volume (FEV) or timed vital capacity, maximum mid expiratory flow rate (MMEFR), peak expiratory flow rate (PEFR), forced expiratory flow at 25%, VC (FEF25) and dynamic compliance.
- Tests of **diffusion** include, lung transfer factor (TLCO), alveolar arterial PO_2 gradient and arterio-alveolar PCO_2 gradient.
- Test for respiratory **control** include: respiratory response to chemical factors like PO_2, PCO_2 and

pH of inspired air and arterial pH, EMG of respiratory muscles.

- **Factors** like respiratory muscle power, airway patency (**resistance**), **compliance** of the lungs and **elasticity** and **viscosity** of lungs, influence **vital capacity.**
- **Vital index** is the vital capacity per sq meter surface area.
- **Breathing reserve** of the lungs is calculated by minusing pulmonary ventilation from maximum voluntary ventilation i.e. BR=MVV–PV.
- **Dyspnoea** means conscious unpleasant breathing or difficulty or labored breathing.
- **Dyspnoea Index** $= \frac{MVV - PV}{MVV} \times 100$ when it falls below 60% there is dyspnoea.
- Examples of **abnormal** respiratory rhythms (periodic breathing) are: **Cheyne stokes** (sleep, hypoxia, heart failure), **Biot's breathing** (brain injury, rise in intracranial tension), **Kussmol** breathing (diabetic ketoacidosis) and **gasping** breathing (premature babies, brain damage).
- Diffusion **coefficient** depends on the **solubility** and **mol weight** of a gas. Compared to CO_2 solubility of O_2 in H_2O is 20 times **less** hence diffusion rate of O_2 is less than CO_2.
- Diffusion coefficients of O_2 is 1.0, CO_2 is 20.3 and CO is 0.81.
- At **high altitude** barometric **pressure** is low (**hypoxia**) at **10,000 ft** hypoxia symptoms start appearing **(hyperpnoea)** and between **15000-18000 ft severe hypoxia** develops and at **20,000 ft** barometric pressure is **50%** of sea level, person may **lose consciousness**.
- **Symptoms** of exposure to **hypoxia** pertains to (a) **CNS** (depression, loss of coordination, easy fatiguability, power of judgement impaired, auditory and visual acuity decreases) as brain is highly susceptible to hypoxia, (b) **respiratory system**

(hyperpnoea and alkalemia, due to washing out of CO_2). (c) **CVS** (tachycardia, rise in BP) and (d) **GIT** (anorexia, nausea, vomiting, diarrhoea, excessive thirst).

- At **sea level**, barometric pressure is **760 mmHg** (1 atmosphere), as person dives into the **depths** of sea, for each **10 meter (33 ft)** depth there is **1 atmospheric** pressure **rise**. At **99 ft** pressure is 3 + 1 = **4 atmospheres.**
- So in deep sea, the diver breathes **hyperbaric gases** and the gases get **dissolved in** tissue fluid at high pressure and cause certain **hazards**.
- Problems of **hyperbarism** or deep sea divers are: (a) **Nitrogen narcosis** (b) **high pressure nervous syndrome** (tremors drowsiness, and lack of coordination) (c) **O_2 toxicity** (nausea, dizziness, irritability, disorientation and disturbed vision, convulsions and coma) (d) **dysbarism** (caisson's disease) from high pressure, subject is brought to sea level suddenly, gas bubbles are formed in blood and tissues.
- Hence **decompression** should be **gradual** should not exceed **50% at a time.**

c. Hypoxia

- **Hypoxia** is a **condition** in which the **metabolic demands** for **O_2 cannot** be met by the **circulating blood.**

  Four principal types of hypoxia are:

  a. **Anaemic hypoxia**—caused by **decrease** in the amount of **Hb available** for **binding O_2**, so that **oxygen content** of **arterial blood** is **abnormally low**.
     - It may be due to **blood loss, abnormal Hb** as a result of genetic defect or **carbon monoxide poisoning** as CO has 250 times more affinity to combine with Hb.
     - The **arterial PO_2** is **normal** but since **O_2 content** of **arterial blood** is **low**, higher

proportion of O_2 is extracted from Hb to **support metabolism**. Consequently **venous PO_2** is much **lower than normal**.

b. **Stagnant hypoxia**—is **due to slow, sluggish blood flow.** May result from **local vasoconstriction (exposure to cold)** or **reduced cardiac output.** In this case **alveolar** and **arterial PO_2** may be **normal, excessive extraction** of O_2 by **tissues reduces PO_2** in **venous blood** to very **low level**—giving rise to peripheral **cyanosis.**

c. **Histotoxic hypoxia** refers to **poisoning** of the **oxidative enzymes** by **cyanide.** Supply of **O_2** to **tissue is normal** but **utilisation is poor** hence **PO_2** is **abnormally high** in **venous blood.**

d. **Hypoxic hypoxia** is due to **exposure to low atmospheric** or **alveolar PO_2** (high altitude or lung diseases).
   - It can be **treated by administration** of **high partial pressure oxygen.**
   - By **increasing** the **partial pressure of O_2** in **alveoli,** the **O_2 content** of the blood **leaving lungs** is **raised.**
   - In **CO poisoning, hyperbaric O_2** (pressure **more than atmospheric)** is **administered.** The high **PO_2** acts to **displace the CO bound to Hb** and provides much needed **O_2 to tissues.**

d. Gaseous Exchange

- In the **steady state,** net volumes of **O_2 and CO_2** exchanged in the lungs per **unit time** are equal to the net volumes exchanged **in the tissues.**
- Typical volumes exchanged per **minute** are, O_2 250 ml and CO_2 **200 ml.**
- **Exchange** of these **gases** in lungs and tissues is by **diffusion** due to difference in **gas partial pressures.**

- Normal PO_2 in alveolar air is **105 mmHg** and for CO_2 it is **40 mmHg**.
- Average value for systemic venous **PO_2 is 40 mmHg** and for **PCO_2, 46 mmHg.**
- As the systemic venous blood flows through the **pulmonary capillaries** there is **net diffusion** of O_2 from alveoli to **blood** and of **CO_2** from blood to **alveoli**.
- By the **end of pulmonary capillary**, the blood **gas pressures** have become **equal** to those in **alveoli**.
- Therefore PO_2 and PCO_2, in the systemic arterial blood are virtually **identical** to **those in alveoli.**
- **Inadequate** exchange between alveoli and pulmonary capillaries may occur, when the capillary **surface area** is **decreased,** alveolar **walls thicken** and when there are **ventilation-perfusion inequalities.**
- Ventilation-perfusion inequalities are **minimised** by **local intrapulmonary** homeostatic response in which the low PO_2 **constricts** the pulmonary blood vessels and the **high PCO_2 dilates** them.
- The major consequences of uncompensated mismatching is that the systemic **arterial PO_2** is considerably **lower** than **alveolar** PO_2.
- In the **tissues** net O_2 **diffusion** occurs from **blood** to **cells** and net diffusion of **CO_2** from **cells** to **blood.**

e. Gas Transport

Oxygen

- Each **litre** of systemic **arterial blood** normally contains **200 ml** of O_2, more than 98% of which is **bound** to **haemoglobin**, and the rest of which is **dissloved** in **plasma**.
- The major determinant of the **degree** to which **haemoglobin** is saturated with O_2 is **blood PO_2.**
- **Hb** is almost **100%** saturated at the normal systemic arterial **PO_2** of **105 mmHg.** The fact

that saturation is more than 90% at **PO_2 of 60 mmHg,** permits relatively normal uptake of O_2 by the blood even if alveolar **PO_2** is **moderately reduced.**

- **Hb** is **75%** saturated at the **normal systemic** venous **PO_2 of 40 mmHg.**
- Thus only **25%** of O_2 has **dissociated** from **Hb** to **tissues**.
- The **affinity** of **Hb** for **O_2** is **decreased** by an increase in **PCO_2, hydrogen ion** concentration and **temperature.** All these conditions exit in the tissues and facilitate **dissociation** of O_2 **from Hb.**
- The affinity of Hb for O_2 is **also decreased** by **erythrocyte DPG** which **increases** in situation associated with **inadequate O_2** supply and helps maintain O_2 **delivery** to the **tissues.**

Carbondioxide

- Each **litre** of systemic **arterial blood** contains **550 ml** of total CO_2, **90%** of which is **bicarbonate**.
- When CO_2 diffuses from tissues to **blood**, 10% remains **dissloved** in **plasma** and RBC, **30%** combines with **deoxy Hb** of RBC forming **carbamino-compounds** and **60% combines** with water **in RBC** to form **carbonic acid,** which then dissociates to yield HCO_3^- and H^+. Most of the HCO_3^- diffuse out of RBC to plasma in **exchange** for Cl^- (chloride shift).
- As venous blood flows through lung capillaries PCO_2 decreases because of CO_2 diffusion.

f. Control of Respiration

- Breathing depends on **cyclical inspiratory** muscle excitation by the **nerves** to the **diaphragm** and **intercostal muscles**.
- This **neural activity** is **triggered** by **medullary** inspiratory **neurons (IC)**.

- Most important **input** to **IC** for involuntary control of **minute ventilation** are from the **peripheral** (carotid and aortic bodies) and **central chemoreceptors**.
- Ventilation is **reflexly stimulated** via the **peripheral chemoreceptors**, by a **decrease** in arterial **PO_2** when decrease is large.
- Ventilation is reflexly **stimulated** via both the **peripheral** and central **chemoreceptors** when **arterial PCO_2** goes **up even slightly**.
- The **stimulus** for this **reflex is** not the increased **PCO_2** itself but the **concomitant** increased **H^+ concentration** in arterial blood and **brain extracellular** fluid (CSF).
- **Potent stimuli** for **peripheral chemoreceptors** are **decreased PO_2** increase in **PCO_2** and **decrease in pH**. The result of these reflexes is to restore H^+ concentration towards normal by **lowering PCO_2.**
- **Ventilation** is reflexly **inhibited** by an increase in **arterial PO_2** and by a decrease in **arterial PCO_2** or **increase** in pH.
- During **moderate** exercise, **ventilation** increases in exact **proportion** to **metabolism,** during very strenuous exercise, **ventilation increases** more than **metabolism**.
- The **proportional increase** in ventilation during moderate exercise cause the **arterial PO_2, PCO_2,** and **H^+ concentration** to remain unchanged.
- Arterial **H+ concentration** increases during **very strenous exercise** because of **increased lactic acid production.** This increase, accounts for some of the hyperventilation seen in that situation.
- **Ventilation** is also **controlled** by reflexes originating in airway receptors, by painful and emotional stimuli and by **conscious intent.**
- Non respiratory functions of lungs include **defence, sieves for small clots** in blood and **removal of toxic** and **absorption** of **medicine** (aerosols).

Chapter Six

GIT Nutrition

a. General Features

- A **balanced diet** is **essential** for **health**. The mixed diet contains **adequate** amounts of the **essential nutrients**.
- GIT, transfers organic **nutrients, minerals** and **water** from external environment to the internal environment.
- The **four** processes used to accomplish this function are, **digestion, secretion, absorption** and **motility** (elimination of waste, non-used products).
- **Carbohydrates** are **absorbed** in form of **mono-saccharides** and they provide **energy.** They may be **stored** in form of **glycogen** or **fats.**
- **Proteins** are broken down into **amino acids** which are absorbed and utilised to make **structure protein, enzymes, hormones.**
- The eight out of **10 essential amino acids** must be **included** in diet.
- **Fat** is an **important** source of **heat** and **energy**. forms **protective layers** and is important **constituent** of **cell membranes.**
- **Certain fatty acids** are called as **essential** as they **can't be** manufactured in the body.
- A **wide variety** of **vitamins** and **minerals** are required for normal **functioning** of **cell. Special absorptive mechanism** are available for absorption of these in **GIT.**
- **Hunger** and **appetite** are important **regulators** of **food intake.**

- **Feeding** and **satiety centres** are located in the **hypothalamus-Lateral hypothalamus** for **feeding** and **ventromedial** for **satiety**.
- The **GI tract absorbs** about **10 L** of **fluid** every **day**.
- The **myenteric plexus** lies **between** the **longitudinal** and **circular** muscle layers of the **GI wall.**
- **Swallowing** is a **complex reflex**, **first** part **is voluntary.**
- The **pH** of **saliva** is **alkaline** and becomes **more alkaline** with **high** HCO_3^- concentration as **secretion rises.**
- **Bolus** in the **oesophagus** moves by a wave of **peristaltic contraction**.
- The saliva **contains enzyme α-amylase** that **digests cooked starch.**
- Nervous control of saliva is more important than hormonal control.
- **Intrinsic factor** is secreted by the **parietal cells.**
- **CCK inhibits gastric secretion** as part of **enterogastric reflex.**
- **Cephalic phase** of the gastric secretion **starts even** before the food reaches the **stomach**.
- The intestinal phase contributes **little** to overall **gastric secretion.**
- During **vomiting,** acid is lost from the stomach and metabolic **alkalosis** is seen with **rise** in **plasma pH.**
- The **most vigorous** mixing **movements** in the stomach take place in the **antral region.**
- **Pancreatic acinar** cells store **proteolytic enzymes** as inactive precursors **(trypsinogen)** to avoid **self digestion**.
- **CCK stimulates** pancreatic secretion **rich** in **enzymes**.
- **Pancreatic juice** contains **enzymes** essential for **protein digestion,** hence in their absence protein utilisation in the body will be **impaired** and **weight loss** will result.

- **Bile** is **concentrated** many times in **gall bladder.**
- **Chylomicrons** are **found** in the **lacteals** after a **fatty meal.**
- **Micelles** are the **aggregation** of bile salts and **fats formed** in the **small gut.**
- They **form** a **stable suspension** that permits digestion of fats **by lipase.**
- **70% blood flow** to **liver** is via **portal vein**.
- **Cystic ducts drain** the **gall bladder**.
- In **obstructive jaundice, faeces** are **clay colored** (pale) and fatty (bulky).
- **Cellulose cannot be digested or absorbed** by the human **small gut**.
- **Gastric acid** is **secreted** by **parietal cells** of the gastric glands.
- The **enzymes** of the **small gut** are **associated** with the **brush borders** of the **epithelial cells.**
- All the **digestion products** of ingested **carbohydrates** are **absorbed in small gut.**
- **Amino acids** are **absorbed** in the **small intestine** by **co-transport with Na^+.**
- The **Na^+, K^+ –ATPase** of the **basolateral membrane** of the intestinal epithelial cells **plays** an **important** role is **absorption** of **salt** and **water.**
- The **first organ** to **receive** the **blood borne products** of **digestion** is **liver.**
- **Intrinsic factor, secreted** by **parietal cells** is needed for the **absorption** of **vitamin B_{12}.**
- **Following gastrectomy, large amounts** of **hypertonic chyme** enters the **duodenum, water** enters the **gut lumen** down the **osmotic gradient,** leaving the **plasma more concentrated.** This is called as **'Dumping Syndrome'.**
- **Parasympathetic** stimulation **enhances intestinal motility.**
- **Distension** of the **ileum inhibits** intestinal **motility** (Intestino-intestinal reflex).

- **Vitamin K** is **required** for **normal blood clotting** hence **bleeding disorders** are seen in its **deficiency.**
- **Vitamin B_{12} deficiency** leads to **pernicious anaemia.**
- **Plant foods do not** contain all the **essential amino acids.**
- **Dietary fibres increase** the **transit time** through **the colon.**
- **Vitamin K synthesis** by the **intestinal bacteria** is important for the maintenance of **normal hemostasis.**
- **Gastrin** facilitates ileal **emptying.**
- **Gastric** and duodenal **ulcers** can be given **a chance** to **heal** by **inhibition** of **acid secretion** by drugs such as **cematidine (H_2 histamine receptor blocker)** or **omeprazole** (inhibit **H^+, K^+, ATPase**).
- The **barrier** in the **stomach** which protects **mucosa** from **HCl action** is **disrupted** by (a) **infection** with **Helicobacter pylori** and (b) use of **nonsteroidal anti-inflammatory** drugs (NSAID).
- These drugs **(NSAID) inhibit** production of **prostaglandins** and consequently decrease **mucus** and **HCO_3^- secretion.**
- Total **plasma bilirubin** normally includes **free bilirubin** plus a **small** amount of **conjugated bilirubin.**
- **Free bilirubin** in **liver cells** is **conjugated** to **glucuronic acid** catalyzed by enzyme **glucuronyl transferase,** to form **bilirubin diglucuronide.**
- Most of the **bilirubin glucuronide** passes via the **bile ducts** to **intestine.**
- **GI hormones** and other **polypeptide** such as **VIP, stimulate secretion** of **intestinal juice.**
- **Resection** of more than **50% of small intestine,** results in **deficit absorption** (malabsorption) leading to **wasting** and **malnutrition.**

- Removal of **small segments** of **jejunum** or **ileum does not** cause **malabsorption** as **compensatory hypertrophy** and hyperplasia of the remaining mucosa looks **after absorption.**
- **Cellulose, hemicellulose** and **lignin** in the diet are important component of **dietary fibres.**
- Each day, GIT secrets about **3.5 times** more fluid into the lumen than is **ingested**. Only about 1% of luminal contents are excreted in faeces.
- The **area** available for absorption in small intestine is **greatly increased** by the **folding** of the intestinal **wall**, the presence of **villi** and the **microvilli** on the surface of the **epithelial** cells.
- The epithelial cells lining the intestinal tract are continuously **replaced** by new cells arising by **mitosis**.
- The **venous** blood from small **gut**, containing absorbed **nutrients** other than fats, passes to the liver via the **hepatic portal vein** before returning to the heart. **Fat** is absorbed into the **lymphatics** (lacteals) in the middle of each **villus**.
- The **enzymes** breaking **proteins** into **peptides** are **pepsin** in the stomach and **trypsin** of pancreatic juice and chymotrypsin of small intestine.
- In small gut peptides are broken down into amino acids by reactions **catalyzed** by pancreatic **carboxypeptidases** and intestinal **aminopeptidases**.
- Large fat globules leaving stomach are **emulsified** in the small intestine by **bile** salts secreted by the liver.
- **Lipase** from the pancreatic juice digests **fats** at the surface of emulsified droplets forming fatty acids and **monoglycerides**.
- These water-**insoluble** products of lipase action, when combined with **bile salts**, form **micelles** that are in equilibrium with free molecules.
- Free fatty **acids** and **monoglycerides** diffuse across the epithelial cells, within which by enzy-

matic recombination action, they **form triglycerides** which are released as **chylomicrons**.

- The **released** chylomicrons enter **lacteals** in the intestinal **villi** and by way of **lymphatics** to the cardiovascular system.
- Water is **reabsorbed** from the small intestine by **osmosis**, following the active reabsorption of **solutes**, primarily **sodium chloride**.
- Most gastrointestinal **reflexes** are initiated by **luminal stimuli, distension, osmolarity, acidity** and **digestion** products.
- Neural **reflexes** are mediated by **short reflexes** in the enteric **nervous** system and by **long reflexes** involving **afferent** and **efferent** neurons to and from the **CNS**.
- **Gastrin**, **secretin**, **CCK** and **GIP** are secreted by **endocrine** cells scattered throughout the epithelium of the **stomach** (gastrin) and **small intestine** (secretin, CCK and GIP).
- The **three phases** of GIT regulation—**cephalic, gastric** and **intestinal** are named after the **location** of the **stimulus** that initiates the response.
- **Salivary** secretion is stimulated by **food** in the **mouth** acting via **chemo** and **pressure**, receptors, both **sympathetic** and **parasympathetic** stimulation increases salivary secretion.
- **Peristaltic** waves sweeping over the stomach become **stronger** in the **antrum**, where most **mixing occurs**. With each wave, only a small portion of the stomach contents are **expelled** into the small intestine through the **pyloric sphincter**.
- The **basic electrical rhythm** (BER) generated by the stomach smooth muscle **determines** peristaltic wave **frequency**. Contraction strength depends on the **frequency** of **action potentials** triggered by the **slow waves**.
- The larger a **meal**, faster the stomach **empties**. Distension of **small gut, fat, acid** or **hypetonic**

solution in the intestinal lumen **inhibit** gastric emptying.

b. GIT Process—Regulation

- The exocrine portion of the **pancreas** secretes **digestive enzymes** and **HCO_3^-**, which reach duodenum through the **pancreatic** duct.
- The **HCO_3^-, neutralizes** acid entering the small intestine from the stomach.
- Most proteolytic enzymes, including trypsin are secreted in **inactive** form. Trypsin is activated by **enterokinase** located on the luminal membrane of small gut and in turn activates other inactive enzymes.
- The hormone **secretin**, released from **small gut** in response to increased **luminal acidity,** stimulates **HCO_3^-**, secretion, while **CCK** is released in response to products **fat** and **proteins digestion** in small gut, stimulates pancreatic enzymes secretion.
- The major ingredients of bile are, **bile salts, cholesterol, lecithin HCO_3^-, bile pigments** and **trace metals**.
- **Bilirubin**, a breakdown product of **haemoglobin** is absorbed from the blood by the **liver** and secreted into the **bile**.
- After reaching small intestine **bile salts** are **reabsorbed** from the **ileum** and travel by **hepatic portal system** to liver (Entero-hepatic circulation).
- The greater the bile **salt concentration** in hepatic portal blood, the greater the rate of **bile secretion**.
- Bile is **concentrated** in **gall** bladder by absorption of bile salt and water.
- Following a **meal**, the release of **CCK** from small intestine causes the gall bladder to **contract** and the sphincter of oddi to **relax**, thereby injecting concentrated bile into the intestine.
- **Hypertonic** solution in the lumen of **small gut inhibits** gastric **motility**.

- Intestinal motility is coordinated by the **enteric nervous** system and **modified** by long and **short reflexes** and **hormones**.
- During and shortly after a meal, the intestinal contents are mixed by **segmental** movements of the **intestinal** wall.
- After most of the food has been digested and absorbed, **segmentation** is **replaced** by the migrating motility complex that sweeps the undigested material into the large intestine by a series of peristaltic waves.
- The primary function of **large intestine** is to **store** and **concentrate** faecal matter.
- In response to **filling, receptive relaxation** of stomach is partly mediated by **vagus nerve**.
- Besides **storing, churning and grinding action and digestion** of food, stomach also produces **intrinsic factor** (for B_{12} absorption), **oxidises ferrous** (Fe^{++}) to **ferric** form. Its acid is **bacteriolytic** and absorption of water, alcohol and saline, to some extent occurs in stomach.
- Gastric secretion is **continuous** and about **1.2–1.5 litres** of juice is secreted/day, during **meals**, secretion is **maximum** and during **sleep** is **minimum**.
- **pH** of gastric juice is highly acidic, i.e. **0.9-1.5**.
- **Contents** of gastric juice are (a) **inorganic** (Na^+, K^+, Cl^-, HCO^-, Ca^{++}, PO^-_4 and HCl). (b) **Organic** (mucus, enzymes, intrinsic factor).
- HCl production in gastric juice is **stimulated** by **vagus, Ach, histamine, gastrin, insulin, caffeine** and **nicotine**.
- HCl production is **inhibited** by **somatostatin, PGE_2, EGF and TGF, Atropine, H_2 blocker, H^+-K^+ pump inhibitors**.
- **Functions** of HCl include: bactericidal agent, activates pepsinogen to pepsin, denaturation of proteins and oxidation of ferrous to ferric state.
- **Gastric** function tests are: (a) **Fractional test meal**, histamine augmentation test, (b) endoscopy,

(c) **barium** meal study (d) **scanning and MRI**.

- The **destruction** of gastric mucosa by HCl is **prevented** by some structures which constitute **gastric mucosal barrier (GMB)**.
- GMB consists of **cell membrane**, **tight junction** between surface epithelial cells, thick **insoluble mucous** over the gastric mucosal cells, **HCO_3^-** secreted by mucosal cells under influence of PGE.
- Besides **storage** and **concentration** of **bile**, gall bladder **converts alkaline** bile to **neutral** bile, secretes **mucin** like material and regulates the **pressure** within **biliary system.**
- **Succus entericus** contains many **enzymes** like **amylase, lipase, peptidases, invertase, isomaltose, lactase, proteases nucleotidases** and **nucleosidases.**
- Four **types** of movements are seen in small intestine; (a) rhythmical **segmental** movements (b) **pendular** movements (c) **peristalsis** (d) **villi** movements.
- Functions of **large intestine** include:
  a. Reservoir for **faecal** matter.
  b. Absorption of substances such as **water, electrolyte, vit. B complex**, some **anaesthetic agents.**
  c. Affects **ECF** volume.
  d. **Synthesis** of various **substances** such as various **vit. B complex** (riboflavin, **nicotinic acid, biotine, B_{12}** and **folic acid**) and **vit. K.**
  e. **Mucus** secretion.
  f. Bacterial **digestion** of **cellulose**, hemicellulose.
- Movements of large intestine include **mixing** movements and **mass** peristalsis.
- **Constipation, diarrhoea,** chronic **ulcerative colitis** and **aganglionic megacolon** are the **disorders** of motility of large intestine.

c. Pathophysiology of GIT

- The factors that normally prevent breakdown of the mucosal barriers (ulcers) are (a) **secretion** of **alkaline** mucus (b) **tight junctions** between **epithelial cells** (c) rapid **replacement** of **epithelial cells**.
- **Precipitation** of **cholesterol** or less often bile **pigments** in the **gallbladder** forms **gall stones**, that can block the exit of gall bladder or bile ducts, leading to (a) **decreased** digestion and absorption of fats (b) **accumulation** of bile pigments in **blood** and tissues (jaundice).
- In the **absence** of **lactase** lactose cannot be digested and its pressure in small intestine retains water, leading to **diarrhoea** and increased **flatus** production **(Lactose intolerance).**
- **Constipation** is probably the result of decreased **colonic motility**.
- **Diarrhoea** is caused primarily by **decreased** fluid **absorption** increased fluid **secretion** or both.

d. Energy Balance—Basic Concepts

- The energy liberated during a chemical **reaction** appears either as **heat** or **work**.
- **Total energy** expenditure = **heat** produced + **external work** done + energy **stored**.
- Basal metabolic rate is increased by **thyroid** hormones and **epinephrine**.
- Energy **storage** as **fat** can be **positive** or **negative** when metabolic rate is **less** than or **greater than,** respectively, the energy content of ingested food.
- Energy storage is regulated mainly by **reflex** adjustment of food **intake** to **metabolic rate.**
- In addition metabolic rate increases or decreases, to some extent when food intake is chronically **increased** or decreased.
- **Obesity,** the result of **imbalance** between food **intake** and **metabolic** rate increases the incidence of **many diseases.**

- Hence **increase** in **waist line** causes **decrease** in **life line.**

e. Fuel Homeostasis in Exercise and Stress

- During **exercise** the muscles use as their **energy** sources plasma **glucose**, plasma **fatty acids** and their **own glycogen**.
- Glucose is produced by the **liver**, and fatty acids are provided by **adipose tissue** lipolysis.
- The changes in plasma **insulin**, **glucagon** and **epinephrine** are similar to those that occur during the **post absorptive** period and are mediated mainly by the **sympathetic** nervous system.
- **Stress** causes metabolic and hormonal changes similar to those of **exercise**.
- **Type 1 diabetes mellitus** is due to absolute insulin **deficiency** and can lead to diabetes **keto-acidosis**.
- **Type 2** diabetes mellitus is usually associated with **obesity** which causes **insulin resistance** and a normal or **even** elevated plasma **insulin** concentration.

f. Regulation of Plasma Cholesterol

- Plasma cholesterol, a precursor for **synthesis** of plasma **membrane bile acids,** and **steroid** hormones, is carried mainly by **low density lipoproteins**, which deliver it to cells, **high-density lipoproteins** carry cholesterol from **cells** to the **liver**.
- The ratio of **LDL/HDL** correlates with the incidence of **coronary disease.**
- Cholesterol **synthesis** is mainly by the **liver** and varies **inversely** with ingested cholesterol.
- The liver also secretes cholesterol into the **bile** and coverts cholesterol to **bile acids**.

Chapter Seven

Renal Physiology

a. General Features

- The kidneys **regulate** the **water, pH** and **ionic** composition (electrolyte) of the body, excrete **waste** products and foreign chemical and **secrete** three **hormones—renin** (angiotensin system), **1,25-dihydroxy vitamins** D_2 and **erythropoietin.**
- Each **nephron** in the kidneys consists of a **glomerulus** and a **tubule.**
- Glomerulus comprises a capillary tuft, which is supplied by an afferent arteriole, and a **Bowman's capsule** into which the **tuft** protrudes.
- The tubule extends out from Bowman's capsule and is subdivided into **four segments,** proximal convoluted tubule (PCT), loop of Henle, distal convoluted tubule (DCT) and collecting duct (CD). The latter empties into **renal pelvis** from which urine flows through ureters to the **bladder**.
- An **afferent** arteriole leaves glomerular capillary tuft and branches into **peritubular** capillaries which supply the tubule.

b. Basic Processes

- The **three** basic renal processes are, glomerular **filtration,** tubular **reabsorption** and tubular **secretion**. In addition, kidneys synthesise or metabolize certain substances.
- Urine formation begins with **glomerular filtration**—approx **180 L/day** of essentially protein free plasma into Bowman's capsule.

- Glomerular filtrate contains **all** the plasma **constituents minus proteins** and substances bound them, in virtually same proportion as in plasma.
- The filtrate is driven by **hydrostatic** pressure in glomerular capillaries and is **opposed** by both the hydrostatic pressure in **Bowman's** capsule and **colloid osmotic** pressure of plasma proteins.
- As the filtrate moves through tubules, certain substances are **reabsorbed** into **peritubular** capillaries.
- Tubular reabsorption **rates** are very **high** for **nutrients, ions and water**, but are lower for **waste products**.
- **Reabsorption** may occur by **carrier-mediated** mechanism or by **diffusion**.
- Many of the carrier-mediated systems manifest **transport maximum** so that when the filtered load exceeds tabular maximum, **large amount** of substances will **escape** reabsorption and appear in **urine**.
- Diffusion occurs for some substances to which tubular **epithelium** is **permeable**, because water reabsorption creates tubule-**interstitium diffusion gradients** for them.
- Tubular **secretion**, movement from the peritubular capillaries into the tubules, is a pathway in addition to glomerular filtration for a substance to gain **entry** to the **tubule**.
- **Micturition** occurs when bladder **distention** stimulates **stretch** receptors that trigger **spinal reflexes** leading to parasympathetically mediated **contraction** of the bladder smooth muscle.
- Voluntary **control** is exerted chiefly by stimulating or inhibiting the nerves to the **pelvic diaphragm**.
- The body **gains** water via **ingestion** and internal **production** (during metabolism) and it **loses** water via **urine**, **GIT** and **evaporation** from the **skin** (of sweat) and respiratory tract.

- For body water and sodium, the major **homeostatic** control point for maintaining stable balance is **renal excretion**.
- Approximately **two-thirds** of the **body water** is in the **intracellular** compartment and **one-third** in **extracellular**. The amount of **sodium** in the body determines the extracellular volume.

c. Reabsorption in Tubules

- **Sodium** is freely filtrable at the glomerulus, and is reabsorbed by primary active process involving **Na^+ K^+ ATPase pump** in the basolateral **membrane** of tubular **epithelium**.
- Sodium reabsorption also drives by **cotransport** the secondary active reabsorption of **glucose, amino acid, chloride** and by **counter transport** the secretion of H^+.
- Sodium reabsorption creates an osmotic gradient across the tubule, which drives water reabsorption of **osmosis**.
- Water reabsorption at late **distal tubules** and **collecting ducts** depends on presence of **ADH**, which increases **permeability** of these tabular segment to water.
- A **large** volume of dilute urine is produced when ADH is **reduced** and therefore water reabsorption is low.
- A small volume of **concentrated** urine is produced by the tabular **counter current multiplier** system when plasma ADH concentration is **high**.
- The **active reabsorption** of NaCl by the **ascending** loop of Henle causes a **progressive concentration** of the **interstitial** fluid of **medulla**.
- The concentrated interstitium causes water to **move out** of the collecting ducts, made highly permeable to water by ADH. The result is **concentration** of collecting duct fluid and the urine.
- Hence urine, **ordinarily** is always **hypertonic** to plasma.

- Sodium excretion in urine is the **difference** between the amount of sodium **filtered** and the amount **reabsorbed**.
- GFR and therefore filtered load of sodium are controlled by **baroreceptor** reflexes. Decreased BP (as in shock) causes decreased **firing** of these receptors, more **sympathetic** out flow to the renal **arterioles**, resulting in **vasoconstriction** and decreased GFR.
- Major control of tubular sodium **reabsorption** is the **adrenal cortical hormone aldosterone,** which stimulates Na^+ reabsorption in the late distal tubule and **collecting** ducts.
- The renin-angiotensin system is one of the major **controllers** of aldosterone secretion.
- Renin is secreted by granulosa cells of JGA, catalyses formation of angiotensin I from angiotensinogen produced by liver. **Converting enzyme** changes it to angiotensin II which stimulates adrenal aldosterone.
- When extracellular volume **decreases**, renin secretion is stimulated by three inputs:
  a. Stimulation of **renal sympathetic** nerves to granular cells by baroreceptor reflexes.
  b. Pressure decrease sensed by the **granular cells** themselves and
  c. A signal generated by **low sodium** or **chloride** concentration in the lumen of the **macula densa**.
- Atrial **natriuretic** factor (ANF) secreted by cells in the atria in response to atrial **distention**, inhibits sodium **reabsorption**.
- Water reabsorption is mainly regulated by ADH, controlled by left atrial **stretch** (baro) receptors and **osmoreceptors** in the **hypothalamus**.
- Via baroreceptor reflexes, **high** extracellular fluid volume **inhibits** ADH secretion and a low volume stimulates it.
- Via **osmoreceptors,** a high body fluid osmolarity stimulates **ADH** secretion and a low osmolarity **inhibits** it.

- Thirst is stimulated by a variety of **inputs**, including **baroreceptors, osmoreceptors** and **angiotensin II.**
- Sodium reabsorption by **aldosterone** results in **potassium secretion**.
- The kidney not only **excretes** H^+ but reabsorbs HCO_3^-.
- Both processes require **tubular** H^+ secretion in a process catalyzed by **carbonic anhydrase**.
- The excreted H^+ is in combination with urinary buffers, probably **ammonia** produced and secreted by the tubules.
- Acid-base **disorders** are categorized as **respiratory** or **metabolic**.
- Respiratory **acidosis** is due to CO_2, and respiratory alkalosis to excessive elimination of CO_2 (washing out).
- All other causes of acidosis, alkalosis are termed **metabolic** and reflect **gain** or **loss**, respectively of H^+ from a **source other** than CO_2.
- **Diuretics** inhibit reabsorption of Na^+ and water thereby enhancing their **excretion** in urine.
- Different diuretic agents act on **different** segments of tubules.
- **Basement** membrane of the glomerular capillary is barrier to the **filtration** of **protein** molecules.
- As per **glomerulo-tubular balance** hypothesis, an **increase** in flow of **tubular fluid** to the **macula densa** will result in **decrease** in GFR.
- Increased oncotic pressure in peritubular capillaries of PCT will enhance **obligatory** water **reabsorption.**
- **Infusion** of **hypertonic** saline would **stimulate ADH** secretion from **posterior pituitary.**
- The **juxtamedullary** nephrons differ from **cortical** nephrons, not only in their **location** and **distribution** but there are a few **functional** differences: Juxtamedullary nephrons **take part** in **countercurrent mechanisms,** flow of filtrate

is **very slow** here, loop of henle are **very long** (thus increasing area for exchange).

d. Methods of Study of Renal Functions

- The methods used to study tubular functions are:
  a. Stop flow technique.
  b. Micro cryoscopic.
  c. Clearance (PAH, inulin, creatinine and urea).
  d. Micropuncture techniques (free flow, stopped flow microperfusion, continuous microperfusion.
- Renal function tests include:
  a. Estimation of blood **urea** and **creatinine** levels (normal urea is 20-40 mg% and creatinine is 0.5–1 mg%).
  b. Examination of **urine** (vol, sp gr, protein, sugar, microscopic and culture).
  c. **Clearance** tests (PAH for blood flow, **inulin** and **creatinine** for **GFR**, urea standard and maximum clearance).
  d. Water **deprivation** test (concentrating power).
  e. Intravenous **pyelography** (IVP) for excretory power of kidney.
  f. Intravenous **radio isotope** renography (blood flow and excretion).
  g. **CAT** and **MRI** scans (for diagnosing various **parenchymal** disorders).
  h. Biopsy.
- Renal failure is defined as deficiency of renal function and it can be (a) **acute** and (b) **chronic** renal failure.

e. Kidney and Homeostasis

- **Urine pH** is normally **much lower** than that of **plasma** and contains **no bicarbonate**.
- If the plasma **pH is elevated (alkalemia)** then the kidneys will excrete **bicarbonate** so that **urine pH rises.**

- **Urine concentration** of **potassium** is **greater** than that of **plasma** (as Na+ reabsorption exchanges for K^+ excretion).
- The **plasma concentration** of **calcium** is **greater** than that of **urine.**
- Urine normally contains **no measurable** quantity of **protein.**
- As **cardiac output rises** in exercise, **renal blood** flow does **not increase**. It **really falls** due to **vasoconstriction activity** of the **sympathetic nerves** to the afferent arterioles (like action on other splanchnic vessels).
- **Para-amino hippuric** acid (PAH) clearance measures renal blood flow (as PAH is filtered as well as secreted by nephrons.
- The **kidneys receive** about a **fifth** of the **cardiac output**.
- **Renal blood flow** is **maintained** within **narrow limits** by **autoregulation.**
- The concentration of **small molecules** in the **glomerular filtrate** is the **same** as in plasma, but the filtrate contains **very little protein** (unlike plasma).
- A **clearance less** than that for **inulin** can be due either to a **barrier** to **filtration** (e.g. plasma proteins) or to **reabsorption** by the **renal tubules** (e.g. glucose).
- The **GFR** can be determined by measuring **clearance** of **inulin** and **creatinine.**
- The **GFR** is **125 ml/min** in adults.
- GFR **depends primarily** on the **pressure** at **afferent arterioles**.
- **Absorption** of most of the **small molecules and ions** in tubules is through **transcellular** route utilising **carrier proteins** or **ion channels**.
- Some of the **molecules** are absorbed through **paracellular route** by **solvent drag** or as a result of **charge difference between** the **lumen** and the **interstitial space**.

- The **appearance** of **glucose** in the **urine** reflects a saturation of the **glucose carriers** of the **proximal tubules.**
- The **GFR** is **closely matched** to the **transport capacity** of the tubules by **glomerulo-tubular feedback.**
- **Tubular** HCO_3^- is converted to CO_2 **and** H_2O by the secretion of H^+ **by an Na+/H+ antiporter** in the **PCT** and H^+ **ion ATPase in the DCT.** It then enters the tubule cells as CO_2 and H_2O where it is **reconverted to** HCO_3^-.
- It passes from the cells to the blood in **exchange for** Cl^-.
- While most of the HCO_3^- is **reabsorbed** in **PCT**, the fluid reaching **DCT** contains about **2 mmols/ L.**
- In the **healthy person, proximal** tubule **reabsorb all the filtered glucose.**
- The **proximal tubules** clear the blood of **bile salts** by **secreting** them into **tubular fluid.**
- There are **15% of juxtamedullary** nephrons and rest are **cortical nephrons.**
- **Juxtamedullary nephrons** have **long loops of Henle** extending deep into **medulla.**
- The cortical nephrons have **small loops,** usually not reaching medulla.
- The **thick ascending limb** of the **loop of Henle transports sodium, potassium** and **chloride** from tubular fluid by a **specific electroneutral carrier.**
- In **PCT,** most Na+ is **reabsorbed** with **small organic molecules or** HCO_3^-.
- The **descending thin limb of loop** of Henle is **permeable to** H_2O.
- The **osmolarity** of the **fluid** at the **hairpin bend** of the loop of **Henle may** exceed **1200 mOsm/ L.**
- The **thin ascending limb** of the **loop of Henle** is **impermeable to water.**
- **Sodium balance** is **regulated** by the activity of **the cells of the distal tubules. Sodium uptake**

by the **PCT** is **obligatory** and linked to absorption of small molecules like Cl– and HCO_3^-.

- **Renin** is an **enzyme**, secreted by the cells of **macula densa in response** to low **sodium** in the fluid **reaching DCT.**
- **Renin cleaves angiotensin I** from a precursor molecule called **angiotensinogen** present in the plasma.
- **Angiotensin I**, gets transferred to **angiotensin II** by the action of **converting enzymes** (AC enzyme).
- **Plasma potassium** is regulated by the **activity of the cells** of the **distal tubules.**
- **Calcium reabsorption** by the cells of the **distal tubule** is increased by **parathormone**.
- **Parathormone** acts on cells of the **proximal tubule** to regulate **phosphate uptake.**
- Without the **buffering action** of **phosphate,** the kidneys would be able to **excrete less than 1 mmol of hydrogen** ions per day.
- The **intercalated cells** of the **distal tubule secrete H^+** to **reabsorb HCO_3^-** from the **tubular fluid**.
- **ADH** is secreted by the **posterior pituitary** in response to an **increase** in plasma **osmolarity**.
- **Following** the **intake** of **large volume** of **water**, a normal person can produce urine with an **osmolarity** of less than **100 mOsm**/L **(water diuresis**).
- The **renal medulla** has an **osmotic gradient** which **increase** from the **border** with **cortex** to the renal **papilla**.
- The **osmotic gradient** in the **medulla results** from the **transport of** sodium **and chloride** ions from the **thick ascending limb of loop** of **Henle** to the **interstitial fluid**.
- ADH acts on **DCT** to increase their permeability to water.
- **Transport maximum for glucose** (TmG) is **360 mg**/min in males and **325 mg**/min in females.

Chapter Eight

Endocrine System

a. Hormones—Structure, Synthesis and Control

- The **amine** hormones are the iodine containing **thyroid hormones** (T_3 and T_4) and the **catecholamines** mainly epinephrine secreted by **adrenal medulla**.
- Most hormones are **peptides** and are synthesized as **larger** molecules that are then **cleaved** .
- **Steroid** hormones are produced from **cholesterol** by the **adrenal cortex** and the **gonads** the **placenta** during pregnancy.
- Most important steroid hormones produced by the **adrenal cortex** are the **mineralocorticoids**. Aldosterone, **glucocorticoids**, cortisol and two **androgens**.
- The **ovaries** produce mainly **estradiol** and **progesterone**, and the **testes** mainly **testosterone**.
- Peptide hormones and catecholamine, **dissolve** in the plasma **water**, but steroid and thyroid hormones, being **water insoluble**, circulate mainly **bound** to plasma **proteins**.
- The **receptors** for the **steroid** and **thyroid** hormones are **inside** the **target** cell, those for the **peptide** hormones and **catecholamines** are on the **plasma membrane**.
- Intracellular receptors activated by **steroid** and **thyroid** hormones combine with **DNA** in the nucleus and induce the **transcription** of DNA into **mRNA**, the result is increased **synthesis** of particular **proteins**.

- **Membrane** receptors activated by **peptide** hormones are **catecholamines,** utilize one or more of the **signal transduction** mechanisms available.
- The **pituitary** gland comprising of anterior and posterior pituitary, is **connected** to the **hypothalamus** by a **stalk** containing **nerve** fibres and **blood vessels**.
- The nerve fibres, which originate from **supra-optic** and **para-ventricular** nucleus of **hypothalamus** and terminate in **posterior pituitary** secrete **oxytocin** and **vasopressin**.
- Secretions of the **anterior** pituitary hormones is **controlled** by **hypothalamic releasing** factors (hormones) secreted into capillaries in the median eminence and reaching the anterior pituitary via the **portal blood**.
- The secretion of each releasing hormone is **controlled** by neuronal and **hormonal inputs** to the hypothalamic neurons.
- Angiotensin II stimulates **zona glomerulosa** of **adrenal cortex** for release of **aldosterone.**
- **Transfer** of cholesterol into **mitochondria** is the **rate limiting** step in synthesis of adrenal cortical **hormones.**
- Besides ACTH, CRH, hypoglycaemia also stimulates cortisol secretion from adrenal cortex.
- Sodium **retention** and potassium **depletion** from plasma is feature of **aldosterone** action on **renal tubes.**
- In comparison to T_4, T_3 has **more affinity** for thyroid **receptors.**
- Secretion of **prolactin** differs from other anterior pituitary hormones, as it is **under tonic inhibition** from **hypothalamus.**
- Amino acid arginine stimulates synthesis and release of **growth hormone.**
- Hypothalamic peptide **hormones** are secreted in a **pulsatile** fashion.

- For each pulse to occur, there is **episodic** increases in **electrical burst** activity in the secretory neurons.
- **Leptin** is synthesised by **adipose** tissue cell and **feeds back** to hypothalamus.
- Steroid hormones are **lipid soluble**, can **alter gene transcription** and are secreted as they are synthesised.

b. Releasing Hormones

- **Hypothalamic** releasing hormones are synthesised and secreted by hypophysiotropic area neurons.
- **Blood flows** from this area to the anterior pituitary gland via the **hypothalamo-hypophyseal portal system.**
- Most of the factors are release stimulating but **prolactin** secretion is controlled by **release inhibiting factor**.
- **Dopamine** acts as a inhibitory hormone on the pituitary lactotrophs that secrete prolactin. Hence loss of **dopamine neurons** in the hypothalamus is likely to lead to a **rise** in **secretion of prolactin**.
- **GH** secretion is under control of both **somatostatin** and **GhRH**.

c. Pituitary Dysfunction

- **Acromegaly** is a disorder characteristic of **hypersecretion** of **GH in adults**.
- **Deficient secretion** of **GH** in **childhood** results in **pituitary dwarfism** in which **body proportions** are **normal**.
- It is **lack** of **ADH** (vasopressin) from the posterior pituitary that increases the risk of **dehydration**.
- **Lack** of **pituitary gonadotropins** (FSH, LH) will lead to delay or **failure of sexual maturation** due to lack of stimulation of gonads.
- Deficient anterior pituitary function in relation to thyroid control will lead to low **TSH** levels and so

thyroid hormone secretion will be depressed leading to reduced **BMR**.

- **Chromaffin cells** are found in **adrenal medulla** as well as in some other locations (small intestine). Epinephrine/Norepinephrine released through them, raise **arterial BP through** their action on both the heart (positive chronotropic and inotropic) and vasculature.
- The **catecholamine release**, increases **heart rate** and **activates lipases** which mobilize fats to increase the production of **free fatty** acids and **glycerol.**
- When **plasma calcium** levels **are normal, PTH** secretion **stimulates bone formation** through its action on **osteoblasts** (cells which secrete bone matrix).
- While **PTH stimulates** calcium absorption by the renal tubules it has **no direct** action on **the gut.** It does, however, **stimulates** the production of **1,25-dihydroxycholecalciferol**, which stimulates **calcium reabsorption** from gut.
- **Low plasma calcium** level stimulates **PTH secretion**, **high level** stimulates secretion of **calcitonin**.
- When **PTH** levels are **elevated, osteoclasts** activity is **stimulated,** which leads to the **demineralization** of **bone** and **release of calcium** into plasma.
- **Oxytocin stimulates** the **ejection of milk** (lactogenesis) from the lactiferous ducts whereas synthesis of milk **(Galactopoiesis)** is controlled by **prolactin**.
- In **absence of ADH, facultative water absorption** in renal tubules **(DCT and CT) suffers,** and large amount of urine is passed out (**diuresis**).
- **Oxytocin** is released in response to **mechanical stimulation** of **suckling at nipple**, while **ADH is** released in **response to increase** in **plasma volume** or **osmolarity**. These are examples of **neuroendocrine reflexes**.

- **ADH exerts** its actions on DCT and CT by binding to G-protein-coupled receptors.
- All **adrenal cortical** hormones are **steroid** in nature.
- **Pituitary ACTH** acts to maintain the **structural** and **functional integrity** of adrenal cortex.
- Hence the **gland involutes** and **atrophies** on **removal of anterior pituitary.**
- **Aldosterone** produced by **zona glomerulosa** of adrenal cortex **regulates** plasma **sodium level** thereby also regulates **total body water.**
- **Cortisol secretion** shows a **circadian rhythm,** secretion is **lowest** around **midnight,** and rises to a **peak** around **dawn,** declines during the course of **the day.**
- **Cortisol** stimulates **glueoneogenesis, maintains rest of glycogen** for use in periods of fasting.
- Thyroid hormones are essential for the **early development** and maturation of the **central nervous system.**
- **Lack** of thyroid hormone in **foetus** and **early neonates** leads to condition called **cretinism** (thyroid dwarf) in which there is **mental retardation (milestones delayed).**
- **Thyroid hormones** stimulate **metabolism** and when they **are low, BMR is reduced.**
- Normal **BMR** is **40 kcal/hr/sq meter surface area.**
- **Thyrotoxicosis** is caused by **overactive gland,** thus high **levels of T_3, T_4** raise BMR and **elevate heart rate.**
- The thyroid gland **avidly takes up iodine** and incorporates it into **thyroglobulin.**
- **Thyroid function tests** include, estimation of **sleeping heart rate, BMR, serum cholesterol, I^{131} uptake, T3, T4, TSH and PBI levels** in blood **and thyroid scan.**
- Any **enlargement** of thyroid gland is referred to as **goitre.**

- **Iodine deficiency goitre** (endemic goiter) is common in some **iodine deficient 'belts'** where iodine has been leached out of the soil by rain so that **food grown** in the **soil is iodine-deficient**.
- **Thyroid dwarf** (cretin) differs from pituitary dwarf as thyroid drawf has **mental retardation, milestone delayed** (smiling, sitting, standing, walking), **idiotic look, large protruding dribbling tongue, pot belly, disproportionate body, oedema, sexual impotency, low BMR, weak muscles.**

  Whereas **pituitary dwarf** has **proportionate body,** with **all other normal** functions except retarded **growth** (dwarfism).
- **Secretion** of **mineralocorticoids** (aldosterone) from zona glomerulosa of adrenal cortex is controlled by **renin-angiotensin system**.
- Patients of **Addison's disease** has **craving** for **salts.** The **exposed skin surfaces** become **pigmented** because of **enhanced** secretion of **MSH of** pituitary, stimulating pigment producing **melanocyte activity**.

d. Glucose—Homeostasis

- **Glucose** is essential **metabolic substrate**, particularly for **CNS**.
- **Plasma glucose** is closely regulated between 4-8 mmol/L by a number of **hormones**.
- These hormones include; insulin, glucagon, glucocorticoids, catecholamines Growth and **thyroid** hormones. All **except insulin** are **hyper glycaemic** in their action.
- Plasma glucose is **determined** by the **balance** between **intestinal absorption, glucose storage** and **synthesis** by the liver, **uptake by** other tissues.
- **Glucose** is stored in form of **glycogen** and synthesized from **noncarbohydrate precursors (gluconeogenesis)** which takes place chiefly in **the liver**.

- Insulin is synthesised by the β **cells of islets of pancreas** in response to **a rise** in **plasma glucose** and **amino acids**.
- Insulin **stimulates** the **uptake** and **utilisation** of glucose by cells, particularly, **liver, adipose tissue** and **skeletal muscles**, thereby causing a fall in the plasma glucose.
- Insulin also **stimulates** both **glycogen** and **protein** synthesis.
- A **lack of insulin** or of **insulin receptors** give rise to **diabetes mellitus** in which there is **hyperglycaemia** leading to **polyurea, excessive thirst** and **weight loss**.
- **Glucagon** is the **most potent hyperglycaemic** hormone secreted by **α-cells** of **pancreatic** islets and it **acts to** promote **release of glucose** into blood.
- **Glucagon** acts as **antagonist** to **insulin** to provide **short term regulation** of plasma **glucose**.
- **Hypoglycaemia** is the **main stimulus** for the secretion **of glucagon** which then stimulates **glycogenolysis, lipolysis** and **gluconeogenesis.**
- During **more** and **prolonged periods** of **fasting,** other **hyperglycaemic** hormones such as **cortisol, catecholamines, GH** and **thyroid hormones** play a more important role.
- Their effects are geared to the **maintenance of glycogen stores, stimulation** of **gluconeogenesis** and **mobilisation** of **fatty acids** and **proteins** to provide other **metabolic substrate** for those tissues enabling to use them. In this way **glucose** is **spared** for **use** by the tissues **totally depending** on it like **brain.**
- In the **absorptive phase** (just after meal), plasma **glucose** is **high, insulin** levels are **high** and the **hyperglycemic** hormones are **inhibited.**
- During this time, **glycogen stores** are replenished and **glucose uptake** and **utilisation** by cells is **high**.

- In the **post absorptive state (3-hours or so** after meal until next intake of food), **counter-regulatory mechanisms** are **initiated,** i.e, levels of **hyperglycaemic hormones are** enhanced and there is increase in metabolism of **fats** and in prolong fasting proteins, so that glucose is spared for use by **CNS.**
- When plasma glucose levels are **high** and cellular **ATP reserves** are **adequate,** glucose **is stored** in the form of **glycogen** and **triglyceride** when level **falls, glycogen** is broken down (**glyco-genolysis**) to liberate **glucose** and glucose is **synthesised** from non **carbohydrate precur-sors (gluconeogenesis).**
- The liver carries out both these processes.
- In **prolonged starvation** excessive **mobilisation of fats** will lead to the production of **ketones in** the **liver.**
- Although some of these are utilized and meta-bolised but **excess ketones** will appear in **plasma** and **urine (ketosis).**
- **Diabetes mellitus** is characterised by **raised plasma glucose**, which leads to **glycosuria** and **osmotic diuresis.**
- As **glucose cannot be utilised effectively** by many cells (absence of insulin), **fats are broken** down to create alternative **source of energy.**
- Because of anti insulin actions of most of the **hyperglycaemic hormones** (cortisol, GH, Thy-roid, catecholamines) **acromegaly, cushing** syndrome and **stress** can result in **diabetes.**
- **Hypoglycaemia** is defined as a blood glucose level below 2-5 mmol/L or 60 mg/100 ml.
- It can result from (a) **overdosage of insulin** in diabetics (b) an **insulin secreting tumor** (c) **lack** of **GH** or **cortisol, (d)** severe **liver disease** (e) very **severe exercise** or inherited defects of **gluconeogenic enzymes.**
- Symptoms of hypoglycamia pertaining to involve-ment of (i) ANS are: hunger, tachycardia, sweating

pallor and anxiety (ii) **altered brain function**: headache, lack of concentration, confusion and coma.

- Body **gains** or **loses** heat by **three** physical processes i.e. **radiation, conduction** and **convection.**
- **Hypothalamically** induced **behaviour responses** to exposure **to cold environment** are those which **preserve heat** and **avoid its** loss-like wearing **woollens, basking** in the **sun** or **fire place, sipping** frequent **hot beverages, slipping** into **centrally heated rooms, sleeping** in **sleep bags** or **using quilts.**
- Behavioural **responses** to exposure to **hot environment** would be those which **facilitate heat loss,** like **wearing minimum clothes,** going to **swimming pool, hilly areas, sipping cold drinks, working** in **AC rooms**.
- Exposure of body to **cold** environment will **initiate mechanisms** which increase **heat production** and **decrease heat** loss. These include **shivering, hunger, increased muscular activity, non shivering thermogenesis** and **increased secretion** of **catecholamines.**
- **Cutaneous vasoconstriction, piloerection, curling up** and **Horripilation** are the **mechanism** which **preserve heat**.
- Body **mechanisms** activated by **heat** are—**increased heat loss** by **cutaneous vasodilation, sweating, increased respiration (panting)** and **decrease heat production** like **anorexia, apathy** and **inertia**.
- **Homeotherms** (warm-blooded) are those **organisms** which **maintain their body temperature constant** despite wide variation of **temperature** in the **surrounding environment. Mammals and birds** are the examples.
- **Poikilotherms** (cold blooded) are those **animals** which **change** their **body temperature** according

to **surrounding environment.** Examples are **amphibia, reptiles, fish.**

- Some **animals** are **homeotherms** with **seasonal poikilothermy.** During extremes of environment, they **libernate** and body temperature falls.
- **Normal value** for the oral temperature is **37°C** (98.6F°). It is 0.5C° **lower than rectal temperature**.
- During exercise, heat produced by **muscular contraction** is stored in body and the **rectal temperature** normally **rises** as high as **40°C**.
- **Hypothermia** is reduction in **core temperature**. Humans tolerate 21-24°C **hypothermia**.

e. Control of Growth

- A bone **lengthens** as **osteoblasts** at the **shaft** edge of the epiphyseal growth plates **convert cartilage to bone** while new cartilage is being laid down.
- Growth **ceases** when the **plates** are completely **converted** to bone.
- The major environmental factors influencing **growth** are nutrients and disease.
- **Malnutritions** during **in utero** life and **infancy** may produce irreversible **stunting**.
- The **adolescent growth spurt** occurs on average about **2 years earlier** in **girls** than boys.
- **Growth spurt** is **not seen** in **pituitary dwarf** unless treated with **growth hormone**.
- **Long bones** grow by addition of **new cartilage** at the **epiphysis** which later becomes **ossified**.
- **Bone mass** virtually becomes **stable** after **puberty**, beginning to fall from around the **age of 40 years**.
- **Lymphoid tissue** has a **greater total mass** in **children**, falling to adult level **after puberty**.
- The **organic matrix** of bone (osteoid) is **secreted** by **osteoblasts**.
- The **shaft** of the long bone is called **diaphysis**.

- The **dividing cartilage** cells are situated in the **inner regions** of the **epiphyseal junction**.
- Bone **remodelling** involves the **resorption of old** bone by **osteoclast** and the **accretion of new** bone which is dependent on **osteoblast** activity.
- The **flat bones** (skull) develop from **fibrous connective** tissue.
- The **long bones** develop by **endochondral ossification** of a **cartilage** model.
- **Complex** crystals of **calcium phosphate (hydroxy appetite)** are the principal **inorganic components** of bone.
- During **foetal life** the **principal** hormonal regulator of **skeletal growth** and **development** is thought to be **thyroxine**.
- **Growth hormone** stimulates the **synthesis** and **secretion** of the IGFs.
- **Normal** circulating levels of **PTH** are required for **osteoblastic** activity and the **secretion** of **osteoid**.
- **Estrogens** and **androgens** secreted in large amount at **puberty** bring about **closure** of the **epiphyses**.
- **Liver cells** are highly regenerative—**no regeneration** in **nerve cell**.
- **Malignant** cells are less differentiated.

f. Hormonal Influences on Growth

- **Growth** hormone is main **stimulus** of **post natal** growth.
- It stimulates release of **IGI-1** from the **liver** and many other **cells**. IGI-1 then acts **locally** or as a **hormone** to stimulate **mitosis**.
- Growth hormone also acts **directly** on cells to stimulate **protein synthesis**.
- Growth hormone secretion occurs mainly during **sleep** and is higher during **adolescence**.
- **Thyroid** hormones stimulate brain development during **infancy** and bone growth during **childhood** and **adolescence**.

- **Insulin** stimulates **growth** mainly during in **utero life**.
- **Testosterone** and **estrogen** stimulate bone **growth** during **adolescence** but also cause **epiphyseal closure**. Testosterone also stimulates **protein synthesis.**
- **Cortisol** in high concentration, **inhibits** growth and **stimulates** protein **catabolism.**

Chapter Nine

Reproduction

a. General Features

- During **spermatogenesis** number of **chromosomes** are **halved by meiosis.**
- The **primary spermatocyte** undergoes **two meiotic divisions** to give rise to spermatids. Hence **mature sperms** are **haploid.**
- At **birth** an **ovary** contains **all** the **oocytes** it will ever have.
- **Mature ovum** undergoes **meiotic division** prior to **ovulation.**
- Following **fertilization** full **complement (diploid)** of **chromosomes** is **restored.**
- **Sertoli cells** synthesise **androgen binding protein** (ABP) in response to **FSH.**
- **Testosterone** produced by **Leydig cells** binds to the **ABP** of **sertoli cells.**
- The **hormone-protein complex** enables the **sertoli cells** to **maintain** the production of spermatozoa.
- **Sertoli cells nurture** the **spermatozoa** until they become **mature sperms.**
- **Spermatozoa** are **derived** from **germ cells** known as **spermatogonia** which lie within the **basal compartment** of the **seminiferous tubules.**
- **Testosterone synthesis** requires both **FSH** and **LH.**
- **Sertoli cells** prevent free **diffusion** of water **soluble substances** between the **seminiferous tubules** and the **blood.**

- The **initial recruitment** of **primordial follicle** into the **pre-antral** phase is **hormonal independent.**
- During the **proantral phase** the **follicle cells** acquire receptors for various hormones **like FSH and LH.**
- The **granulosa cells** develop **receptors** for FSH and estrogen.
- The **theca cells** acquire receptors for **LH.**
- **Period** before **ovulation** is **follicular phase** and after ovulation is **luteal phase.**
- Ovulation occurs at **mid cycle** i.e. **day 14**—prior to ovulation there is **LH surge.**
- The **luteal phase** is associated with a **large increase** in plasma **progesterone.**
- The **myometrium proliferates** under the influence of **estrogens.**
- The cells of the **theca interna** secrete mainly **androgens,** which are **converted** to **estrogens** by **granulosa** cells in response to FSH.
- After **ovulation,** follicle **collapses** around a blood **clot** to form the **corpus luteum.**
- If **no fertilization** occurs, the **corpus luteum regresses** to form **corpus albicans** which has no **secretory** function.
- In the **absence** of **receptors** for **FSH** and **LH, pre-antral** follicles show **atresia.**
- **Progesterone promotes** full development of the **endometrium.**
- If **no egg** is **fertilized,** progesterone levels **fall** and this is the trigger for **menstruation.**
- **Hence,** in other words, **bleeding** at the **end of** the **menstrual cycle** is known as **'withdrawl bleeding'** (withdrawl of support of progestogen).
- The **main action** of **contraceptive pill** is to **inhibit** pre-ovulatory **LH surge.**
- **LH surge** is an example of **positive feedback,** at **mid cycle** peak level of **estrogen** triggers **LH surge.**

- During **first trimester** of **pregnancy, corpus luteum** is maintained by **Human chorionic gonadotropin** (HCG).
- Presence of **HCG** in the **urine** forms the basis of **pregnancy test.**
- **'Agglutination inhibition'** is the indication of pregnancy in **immunological** tests.
- In **males** gonadotropin secretion is **noncyclic**, but in **post-pubertal females,** an **orderly, sequential** secretion of **gonadotropins** is necessary for the occurrence of **menstruation, pregnancy** and **lactation.**
- In female **GnRH** (Gonadotropin releasing hormone) secretion is **pulsatile. Every pulse** coming after **60-80 mins** and **lasts for 10 min.**
- **Continuous** secretion of **GnRH results** in central **infertility** in **female.**
- Sperms contain **either X** or **Y chromosomes,** whereas ovum contains **X chromosomes.**
- If **Y sperm** fertilises **ovum,** XY pattern results and zygote develops into **genetic male.**
- When **ovum** is fertilised with X **chromosome**, XX pattern and a genetic **female results.**
- In normal cells, the **inactive X chromosome condenses** and can be seen in various types of **cells**, usually near the **nuclear membrane** as the **Barr body,** also called as **sex chromatin**.
- Thus there is a **barr body** for **each X chromosome** in **excess** of **one in the cell.**
- In a **normal female foetus,** the **mullerian duct** system develops into uterus and fallopian tubes. In a normal **male** foetus, the **wolffian duct** system develops into epididymus and vas deferens.
- In **Turner's syndrome**, chromosomal pattern of an individual is XO. Individuals with XXY are males with more incidence for mental **retardation** and the syndrome is called as **Klinefelter's** syndrome.
- XXX (super female) pattern is next in frequency to XXY.

- The YO combination is probably **lethal**.
- Sidinafil **(viagra) inhibits** breakdown of **cGMP** by phosphodiesterase, can be used for **impotency.** Besides **sex chromosomes,** abnormalities may occur in autosomes-non disjunction of **chromosome 21 produces** trisomy **(Down's syndrome)** or mongolism. It is a pure case of autosomal gene excess.
- **Puberty** is defined as the **period** when the **endocrine** and **gametogenic** functions of the gonads **first developed** to the point where **reproduction** is possible.
- In **girls,** the first event is **thelarche,** the development of **breasts,** followed by **pubarche,** the development of **axillary** and **pubic hairs** and then by **menarche,** the first **menstrual period.**
- In **pre-puberal period, gonadotropin** secretion is **not being held** in check by the **gonadal hormones.**
- **Time** of puberty in girls is **8-13 yrs** and boys **9-14 years of age.**
- **Onset of pulsatile secretion** of **GnRH** brings on **puberty.** During period from birth to puberty, a **neural mechanism** is **operating** to **prevent** the normal **pulsatile release** of GnRH.
- The human ovaries become **unresponsive** to **gonadotropins** with **advancing age,** and their function **declines** so that **menstrual cycles disappear**—this is called **menopause.**
- In **women,** the menses usually **become irregular** and **cease** between the age of **45-55 years.**
- **Sensations** of **warmth** (hot flashes), **night sweats** and **various psychic symptoms** are common in **postmenopausal** stage.
- The **normal sperm count** is **80-200 million**/ml, average being 100 million/ml. Less than **20 million** is **abnormally low.**
- If **two** of the **three sperm values** are low, the male is **infertile** (count < 20 million, abnormal sperms >20% and immotile sperms >50%).

- **Erection** of penis is a **parasympathetic phenomenon**. On stimatation of 'nervi erigentes', **acetyl choline, vasodilator substances** like **VIP** and **Nitric Oxide** are released. They act through **cGMP** to cause erection.

b. Male Reproductive Physiology

- The **testes** produce **sperms** in the **seminiferous** tubules and secrete **testosterone** from the **leydig cells.**
- The **meiotic** division of spermatogenesis results in each sperm containing **23 chromosomes**, compared to the original **46 of** the spermatogonia.
- The developing **germ cells** are intimately associated with the **sertoli cells** which perform many functions like **support, nutrition** and **secrete** luminal fluid including **androgen binding protein** and **inhibin** (feed back for FSH secretion).

c. Sperm Transport

- From seminiferous tubules, the sperms pass through the **epididymus,** where they **mature** and are **concentrated**.
- The epididymus and **vas deferens store** the sperm, and the seminal vesicles and **prostate** secrete **bulk** of the **semen**.
- **Erection** of the penis occurs because of vascular **engorgement** accomplished by **relaxation** of the **arterioles** and passive **occlusions** of the vein.
- **Ejaculation** includes **emission**—emptying of semen into the **urethra,** followed by **expulsion** of the semen from the urethra.

d. Control of Male reproduction

- **Hypothalamic GnRH** stimulates **FSH and LH** of anterior pituitary, which then act on the **sertoli cells** to stimulate **spermatogenesis** and **inhibin secretion**.

- Testosterone exerts a **negative feedback** inhibition on both **hypothalamus** and **anterior pituitary** to reduce LH secretion.
- **Inhibin** exerts **negative** feedback on **FSH** secretion.
- Testosterone acting **locally** (**paracrine** influence) on the **sertoli cells**, is essential for **maintaining** spermatogenesis.
- Testosterone also maintains **accessory reproductive** organs and male **secondary** sex characters and stimulates **growth of** muscles and **bone**.
- In many **target** cells, testosterone first undergoes **transformation** to **DHEA** or in the brain to **estradiol**.

e. Female Reproductive Physiology

- The female **gonads**, ovaries produce **ova** and secrete **estrogen, progesterone, inhibin** and **relaxin**.
- The **follicle** surrounding the ova consists of **inner** layer of **granulosa cells** and **outer** layers of **theca** cells.
- At the **beginning** of each menstrual cycle, **several** follicles begin to **develop** into **antral follicles,** but soon only the **largest** (dominant) **follicle** continues its development to **full maturity** and **ovulation.**
- **Following** ovulation, the **remaining cells** of the **follicle** are transformed into **corpus luteum** which lasts about **10 days** to **14** days, if **pregnancy does not** occur.
- The **menstrual cycle** can be **divided,** according to **ovarian events,** into **follicular** and a **luteal phase,** which are approximately **14 days** separated by **mid cycle** LH surge and ovulation.
- During intrauterine life, one X chromosome (and no y chromosome) is essential for development of normal female genital tract and external genitalia.

- **Unlike** production of **ova, spermatogenesis** occurs **throughout** life.
- Human chorionic gonadotropin **maintains corpus luteum** for **initial part** of pregnancy which produces **progesterone.**
- One thing is **common** between **sertoli** and **granulosa** cells that both are **stimulated** primarily by **FSH.**
- Increased insulin resistance is seen in mothers during **last trimester** of pregnancy.
- The **three indicators** of **ovulation** are, rise in **BBT**, **Fern like pattern** of **cervical mucus** and its **skipbarkeit effect.**
- **Natural** contraceptive method for a **young married** couple is **safe period.**
- Three features i.e., **involution** of corpus luteum, **throttling** of the blood vessels of endometrium (due to lack of progesterone support) and **onset** of menstrual **bleeding**, are seen at the end of luteal phase of ovarian cycle.

f. Control of Ovarian Function

- During **early** and **middle follicular** phases, **FSH stimulates** the **granulosa cells** to proliferate and secrete estrogens, and **LH stimulates** the **theca cells** to proliferate and secrete the **androgens** that granulosa cells use to make **estrogens**.
- The **estrogen** exerts **negative** feed back on the hypothalamus and **anterior pituitary** to **inhibit** secretion of **GnRH** and **gonadotropins**.
- During the **late follicular** phase, plasma **estrogen becomes** high enough to elicit **surge** of **LH, which then causes, via** the **granulosa cells,** completion of oocyte's first **meiotic** division and cytoplasmic maturation and **ovulation** and formation of **corpus luteum**.
- During the **luteal phase,** under influence of **small LH,** the corpus luteum secretes **progesterone** and **estrogen**.

- **Regression** of **corpus luteum** results in **cessation** of these hormones.

g. Uterine Changes in the Menstrual Cycle

- The **ovarian** follicular phase is **equivalent** to the uterine **menstrual** and **proliferative** phase, the first day of menstruation is the first day of menstrual cycle.
- The ovarian **luteal phase** is equivalent to uterine **secretory phase.**
- Menstruation occurs when the plasma **progesterone** and **estrogen** levels **fall** as a result of the **regression** of **corpus luteum**.
- During the **proliferative phase, estrogen** stimulates **growth** of the **endometrium** and **myometrium** and causes the **cervical mucus** to be readily **penetrable** by sperm **(thin copious, fern like pattern).**
- During the **secretory** phase, **progesterone** converts the **estrogen primed endometrium** to a **secretory tissue** and makes **cervical mucus** relatively **impermeable** to sperm (**thick, mucus plug**).

h. Puberty

- During **onset of puberty, hypothalamic—pituitary gonadal** chain of **hormones** becomes **active** due to **change** in **brain** function that **permits** increased **secretion of GnRH.**
- In **girls, first sign** of puberty is **either** the beginning of **breast development,** or appearance of **pubic hair.**
- In boys it is **acceleration** of growth of **testes** and **serotum**.
- Like **menopause** in **female** (Cessation of menstrual cycle) there is **no such** thing in **male,** lowered steady **decrease** in **testosterone** is seen after **age** of **40 years**.

i. Fertilisation

- **Fertilisation** occurs normally in **one of the fallopian tubes.**
- Since the **ovum** is believed to be **viable** only for **12-24 hours** after ovulation, **fertilisation** must take place **within this period.**
- Sperms must **undergo** the **acrosome reaction** before they can fertilise the **egg.**
- The fertilized egg is also known as **zygote**.
- **Following** fertilisation the egg completes its **second meiotic division.**
- The **fertilized egg** secretes **HCG** to maintain **corpus luteum.**
- The **placental barrier** is **relatively thick** and impermeable.
- This **prevents foetal proteins** passing into **the maternal circulation** and eliciting **immune response.**
- While **blood gases cross placental** barrier by **passive diffusion, glucose** and **amino acids** pass from mother to foetus by **carrier-mediated facilitated diffusion.**
- The **PO_2** of the **umbilical vein** blood is about 4.25 kPa **(32 mmHg)** which is much lower than PO2 in the **uterine artery** with is 12-6 kPa **(95 mmHg).**
- The **placenta nourishes** foetus by establishing a **dialysis pattern** for exchange between the maternal and foetal circulation.
- The placenta **secretes** about **10 times**. as much **progesterone** as the corpus luteum.
- **Parturition** is an **integrated multifactorial** process **involving diverse mechanisms** in both the **maternal** and **foetal neuroendocrine systems.**
- **Amenorrhoea** is the **absence** of menstrual **periods**. Physiological condition where prolonged amenorrhoea is seen, is normal pregnancy.
- If menstrual bleeding has never occurred, the condition is called as **primary amenorrhoea**.

- **Cessation** of cycles in a woman with previously normal periods is called **secondary amenorrhoea**.
- The **hypothalamic amenorrhoea** is due to **slowing** of GnRH pulsatile rhythm, may be due to excessive opioid activity.
- In such cases **frequency of GnRH pulses** has been improved by administration of **opioid blocking drugs** like **naltrexone**.
- The terms **hypomenorrhoea** and **menorrhagia refer to scanty** and **abnormally profuse** menstrual flow respectively, during regular period.
- **Metrorrhagia** is bleeding from uterus **between periods**.
- **Dysmenorrhoea** is painful menstruation.
- Most of the symptoms of dysmenorrhoea are due to **accumulation** of **protaglandins** in uterus, **inhibitors** of protoglandin synthetase give relief to symptoms.
- The **premenstrual syndrome** (PMS) is referred to symptoms like irritability, bloating, oedema, emotional lability, depression headache and constipation during last 7-8 days of their menstrual cycle.
- **PMS** has been attributed to **salt** and **water retention**.
- The **blastocyst** is **implanted** in the uterus after it takes 3 days to reach it from fallopian tube—by that time it is **8-12 cell stage.**
- **Placental hormones** are: HCG, HCS, HPL Progesterone, estrogens.

j. Pregnancy

- After **ovulation,** the ovum is **swept** into **uterine tube**, where **sperm** having undergone, **capacitation** and **activation** in the female tract **fertilizes** it.
- Following **fertilization,** the **ovum** undergoes its **first meiotic** division, and the nucleus of ovum and **sperm fuse. Reaction** in the ovum **blocks**

penetration by other **sperms** and **trigger** cell **division** and **embryogenesis**.

- The **trophoblast** gives rise to the **foetal part of the placenta,** whereas **inner cell mass** develops into the **embryo.**
- Although they **donot mix, foetal** and **maternal blood** both flow through the **placenta,** exchanging **gases, nutrients** and **waste products**.
- **Human chorionic gonadotropin** produced by **trophoblast** maintain corpus luteum for **first 2-3 months** of **pregnancy**, producing **estrogen** and **progesterone**.
- During **last 6-7 months** of pregnancy, **placenta** itself produces large amount of these hormones.
- The **high** levels of **estrogen, progesterone** inhibits **hypothalamic GnRH** and **pituitary gonadotropin** secretion, resulting in **elimination** of menstrual cycle.
- **Parturition** occurs by **rhythmical** contractions of the **uterus**, which first **dilate** the **cervix** and then move the **foetus** followed by **placenta** through **birth canal.**
- Uterine contractions are **stimulated** by **decrease** in the **progesterone** to **estrogen ratio** (progesterone inhibits, estrogen stimulates), by **oxytocin** released from **posterior pituitary** in a **reflex triggered** by uterine **mechano receptions,** and **prostaglandins.**
- The **breast** develops **markedly** during **pregnancy** as a result of **combined** influences of **estrogen, progesterone, prolactin** and **placental lactogen.**
- As a result of the **suckling reflex, large bursts** of **prolactin** and **oxytocin** occur during **nursing,** the **oxytocin causing** milk **ejection** (let down).

k. Lactation

- After **delivery, milk secretion** is maintained by **regular suckling** (suckling reflex).

- The **hormone** responsible for **galactopoiesis** is **prolactin**, secreted in direct response to **nipple stimulation.**
- Milk **'let-down'** and **milk ejection** are the processes by which milk is **moved** from the **alveoli** of the mammary gland to the **nipple**.
- This **occurs** in response to **oxytocin** secreted by the **posterior pituitary** during **suckling**.
- Once the **baby** is **weaned**, and the **suckling stimulus** is **lost**, prolactin output falls. **Lactation slows** and **ceases altogether 2 or 3 weeks** after the **stoppage of suckling**.
- The nature of prolactin **inhibiting hormone** secreted by hypothalamus is **dopamine**.
- Hence **dopamine agonist** will **suppress prolactin** secretion and milk production.
- **Colostrum** has a **higher proportion** of **protein** content than mature milk but has a **lower fat** and **carbohydrate content**.
- It, therefore has a **lower calorific value** than **mature milk**.
- The **mammary gland** is **prepared** for lactation **early** in **pregnancy** so that **loss** of **placental steroid** hormones will **initiate lactation.**
- During pregnancy **estrogens** stimulate **ductal development** while **progesterone** stimulates **development of the alveoli**.
- Following a **miscarriage** at 5 month's gestation, **lactation** will **commence**, since inhibiting action of **placental steroid** hormone is gone.
- Placental steroid **hormones inhibits** lactation during **pregnancy**.
- **Normal** functioning of the **feto placental** unit is very important for **progress** of **pregnancy** and **well being** and **growth of foetus.**
- **Post-maturity** (delivery beyond 40 weeks) is **indicative** of **reduced** functioning of **feto-placental unit**.

I. Foetal and Neonatal Physiology

- The **blood** in the **umbilical vein** is about **80% saturated** with O_2.
- **Foetal blood** has a **higher haemoglobin** content than adult blood.
- **Foetal haemoglobin** has a **higher affinity** for **O_2** than **adult haemoglobin**.
- The **oxygen content** of blood in **umbilical vein** is about **16 ml/100 ml.**
- As the **blood perfusing** the **foetal brain** is **supplied** via the **ascending aorta** and ductus arteriosus supplies **deoxygenated blood** to the **descending aorta**, the blood perfusing the **brain** has **higher PO_2** than that in descending aorta.
- Most of the **blood** returning in **umbilical vein** passes **directly to** the **left atrium** via the **foramen ovale**.
- **Foetal BP** is normally low 70/45 mmHg (9/6 kPa).
- The **three foetal shunts close** within few **days of birth.**
- The **foetal heart rate** is **nearly double** that of a **healthy adult.**
- The **ductus arteriosis** carries blood from the **pulmonary artery** to the **descending aorta**.
- Very **large pressure** changes **(intra thoracic)** are **required** to **establish breathing** in **neonates**. Hence **lung compliance** is **very low** compared to the adult.
- To **inflate** the **lungs** for the first time, the **neonate generates** a **very large negative intra thoracic** pressure (about 10-15 times the pressure needed for normal inspiration in adult).
- To **exhale** the **first breath**, neonate requires a **large positive intrathoracic** pressure.
- At birth **central chemoreceptors** are **active** and **peripheral** chemoreceptors **become sensitive** in the **weeks following birth**.
- After the **first breath**, the proportion of **right ventricular output** going to lungs, **increases** but

all the blood from right ventricle goes to lungs as **ductus arteriosus closes**.

- **Surfactant** is a **lipid-surface tension lowering** agent.
- It is a **mixture** of dipalmitoyl phosphatidyl choline **(DPPC)**, other **lipids** and **proteins**.
- **Lack** of **surfactant** in the neonate may cause respiratory distress **syndrome (RDS of newborn)**.
- The foetal zone of **adrenal gland** synthesises **large amounts** of estrogen pre-cursors which are converted to estrogen by **placenta**.
- Foetal **cortisol** stimulates the production of **pulmonary surfactant** by alveolar **type II cells**.
- The foetal **kidneys** produce a **hypotonic urine** after about 8 weeks of gestation.
- The **kidneys** play an important role in the **regulation** of **acid-base** balance of the foetus.
- The **neonate** is unable to **generate** very much heat by **shivering**, instead it utilises **non-shivering thermogenesis**.
- Much of this **additional heat** is generated by the **metabolism** of **brown fat**.
- The development of the **foetal gonads** into the **male type** depends on presence of **testosterone**.
- The **sex** of the **individual** is **determined** by a single gene on the **Y chromosome**.
- In the absence of a **Y chromosome** the development of the gonads will follow the **female pattern**.
- Androgens from the foetal testes play important role in **stimulating** development of **internal male genitalia** from the **wolffian ducts**.
- In the presence of **ovaries**, the **Mullerian ducts** develop into **fallopian** tubes, **uterus, cervix** and **upper vagina**.

Chapter Ten

Nerve Muscle Physiology

a. Nerve Fibres

- The nerve **conduction velocity** is affected by various **factors** like, temperature, hypoxia, pressure on nerve, diameter of nerve fibre, myelination, and certain drugs and ions.
- The rule of thumb in determining nerve conduction in **myelinated fibre** is **diameter** (in μm) × **6 M/sec**.
- The **compound action potential** is a **multipeak** action potential recorded from **stimulation** of **mixed nerve**, the **first peak** belongs to the **fastest conducting** fibres (large diameter) and the **last peak** to the **slowest** conducting fibres.
- **Erlanger and Gassier** classification of nerve fibres is based on **diameter** of nerve fibres and **conduction velocity**.
- Based on these, **three** types of fibres are present, **A** with **diameter** 4–20 μm, velocity 24-120 M/sec, **B** with **diameter** 1-3 μm, velocity 6-18 M/sec and **C** with **diameter** < 1 and < 6 M/sec.
- **Type A** is further divided into Aα (diameter 12-20 μm), Aβ (5–12 μm), Aγ (3–6 μm) and Aδ (2–5 μm).
- Afferents or sensory nerve fibres are **classified** as four groups i.e., **group Ia** (muscle spindle, primary annulospiral endings), IB (Golgi tendon organ), **group II** (muscle spindle, secondary flower spray endings, touch, pressure), **III** (pain, temperature, some touch) and **group IV** (pain and other receptors).

- The **degenerative** changes in cell **body (soma)** due to **nerve injury** include disintegration of nissl granules (chromatolysis), disappearance of golgi apparatus, mitochondria and neurofibrils. The cell draws in fluid and swells up, nucleus is pushed to one side or extruded.
- Neurotropins are proteins which stimulate growth and maintenance and functional integrity of neurons. They are produced by muscles, Schwann cells, astrocytes, liver and platelets.
- Some important neurotropins are: Nerve growth factor, insulin like growth factor, fibroblast growth factor, platelet derived growth factor, leukaemia inhibitory factor, neurotropin 3, 4 and brain derived neurotropic factors.
- Main functions of neurotropins include, growth and functional integrity of neuron, prevent cell death (apoptosis), stimulate regeneration of nerve fibre, participate in neural plasticity.
- Their deficiency leads to development of variety of degenerative disorders of neurons.

b. Muscle

- **Troponin** is present in a **1:1 molar ratio** with **tropomyosin**.
- **Fine gradation** of force of muscle contraction is facilitated by the **large number** of **motor units** with relatively few cells.
- As compared to **fast** (white) muscle fibres, **slow** have more **mitochondria**, **blood supply** and **myoglobin content**.
- **Gradation** of force of contraction in skeletal muscle mostly depends on **recruitment** of motor units.
- Excellent performance in long distance running (Marathan) involves contraction of mainly **slow motor units**.
- **Glycolysis** is characterised by **rapid** rates of **ATP synthesis**.

- The **force generated** per cross-sectional area of a smooth muscle is **smaller** to that of **skeletal muscle**.
- **Sarcolema** is responsible for regulating the **myoplasmic Ca^{++}** concentration during **sustained contraction** in smooth muscle.
- In a **relaxed muscle**, the **cross bridges** are a high energy **complex** of **myosin, ADP and P_1**.
- When work is done on a contracting muscle by **external force, cross bridges** are **broken** without **ATP hydrolysis**.
- **Transverse tubular depolarisation does not** occur during initial **Ca^{++} transient** induced by **excitatory** neurotransmitter in **smooth muscle**.

c. Skeletal Muscle

- Skeletal muscles have **cylindrical** muscle **fibres** linked to **bone** on each side by **tendon**.
- These muscles have a **repeated striated pattern** of **light** and **dark bands** due to location of thick and **thin filaments** within the **myofibrils**.
- **Actin** containing **thin** filaments are **anchored** to the **Z lines** at each and of the **sarcomere** (functional and structural unit of muscle). While their free ends **partially overlap** the **myosin** containing **thick filaments** in the **A band**.
- Muscle **fatigue** is caused by internal **changes** in **acidity, glycogen depletion** and **excitation contraction coupling failure** and **not** by lack of ATP.
- There are **three types** of skeletal muscle fibres, **slow oxidative** (red fibres), **Fast oxidative** (tonic) and fast **glycolytic fibres** (white).
- Fast glycolytic fibres (pale or white fibres) have a **larger average** diameter than oxidative fibres and therefore produce **greater tension**, but **fatigue rapidly**.
- **All** the muscle **fibres** in a single **motor unit** are the **same fibre** type and most **muscle** contain all **three fibres** types in **different proportions.**

- Muscles that produce **delicate movements** (extra ocular muscle) have a **small number** of fibres per **motor unit** (small motor units) whereas postural muscles (back and limb muscles) have much **larger motor** units.
- **Slow oxidative** motor units are **recruited first,** followed by **fast oxidative** and **finally** fast **glycolytic** motor units.
- Increasing motor unit recruitment increases the **velocity** at which a muscle will move a given **load**.
- **Long duration, low intensity exercise (Marathan runner) increases fibre's oxidative capacity** for ATP production by increasing the **number** of **mitochondria** and **blood flow** to the muscle, resulting in **increased endurance.**
- **Short duration, high intensity** exercise (100 meter dash) **increases fibre diameter** due to increased **synthesis** of **actin and myosin** resulting in increased **strength**.
- Movement **around** a **joint** requires **two antagonistic** groups of muscles, one group flexes the limb at a joint and the other extends the limb.
- When skeletal muscle fibres **actively shorten**, the **thin filaments** are **propelled towards** the **centre** of each **sarcomere** by movements of the **myosin** cross **bridges** that bind **to actin** on the **thin filaments**.

d. Smooth Muscles

- All muscle cells have actin and myosin proteins.
- **Smooth muscles** consists of **sheets containing** many **small, spindle shaped cells, linked together** at **specific junctions**.
- Smooth muscle cells contain **actin** and **myosin** but these proteins are **not arranged** in **regular sarcomeres.**
- Each smooth muscle cell has **a loose matrix** of **contractile proteins,** that is **attached** to **plasma membrane** at the **junctional complexes** between **neigbouring cells**.

- **Bozler's classification** of smooth muscles is based on their **response to stretch** or **autorhythmicity**—classified into (a) **unitary** (visceral) (b) **multiunitary.**
- **Single unit** smooth muscles show **myogenic activity** and behave as **syncytium**—develop **tension** on **stretching.**
- **Multiunit smooth** muscle has **no or little spontaneous activity** and is activated by stimulation of **specific motor nerves.**
- Both types of smooth muscles are **innervated** by fibres of the **autonomic nervous system.**
- **Steady level** of smooth **muscle tone** may be altered by circulating **hormones,** second messengers or by **local factors** or by **activity of autonomic nerves.**
- Smooth muscle is much more **plastic** and is able to **adjust** its **length** over a much **wider range** than **skeletal** or **cardiac muscle.**
- Skeletal and cardiac muscles are both **striated** but the organisation of each differs considerably.
- Skeletal muscle fibres are large, multinucleated cells with a well developed T. system. Unlike cardiac muscle, individual skeletal fibres are not coupled together via gap junctions.
- In skeletal and cardiac muscle, **actin** is the major protein of **thin** filaments.
- The myofibrils of skeletal muscles are surrounded by the sacroplasmic reticulum.
- The **sacroplasmic reticulum** acts as a **store** of **calcium** for the contractile process and muscle relaxes when Ca^{++} is pumped out.
- A **rise** in **intracellular calcium** allows **actin to interact with myosin.**
- **Calcium entry** across **plasma membrane** is important in **sustaining** the **contraction** of the **cardiac muscle.**
- **Skeletal** muscle fibres **act independently** of each other, **unlike cardiac** and **smooth muscle** cells, which are linked by **gap junctions.**

- **Skeletal muscle** contracts by about **one fifth** of its **resting length. Smooth muscle** can contract by more than **two-thirds** of its **resting length.**
- A **motor unit** consists of a **single motor fibre** and the **muscle fibres** it **innervates**.
- **Postural group of muscles** have **larger sized motor** unit each **motor fibre supplying many muscle fibres.**
- **Peripheral muscles** concerned with **fine, skilled movements** (like extraocular muscles, thumb muscles) have **very small motor unit.** Each **motor fibre** supplying **very few muscle fibres.**
- The **muscle action potential** is an **essential step** in **excitation-contraction coupling.**
- The **energy** for muscular **contraction** comes from **hydrolysis** of **ATP**.
- In the **heart,** while the **myocytes** of the **SA node** generate **spontaneous action potentials** that set the heart rate, all myocytes can **generate pacemaker** and **action potentials.**
- The **heart rate** is **increased (positive chrono-tropic effect)** by **stimulation of** the **cardiac sympathetic** and **inhibited** (negative chrono-tropic) by stimulation of **vagus nerve**.
- The **cardiac action potential** is **much longer than that of** skeletal muscle and has **many phases (0-4).**
- Much of the **calcium required for contraction enters** a myocyte **during** the **plateau phase** of **action potential.**
- The action potential in heart **spreads** from **cell to cell** via **gap junctions.**
- The **force of contraction** of heart is **increased (positive inotropic** effect) by **circulating epine-phrine** or **stimulation of cardiac sympathetic nerve.**

Chapter Eleven

Nervous System

a. General Features

- Nervous system is divided into two parts:
  a. Central Nervous System (CNS) comprising brain and spinal cord.
  b. **Peripheral Nervous System (PNS)**, consisting of **nerves** extending from periphery to **CNS**.
- **Basic** unit of nervous system in nerve cell or **neuron**, its **soma** (cell body) and **dendrites** receive information from other cells, whereas **axons** transmit information.
- The **axon** (nerve fibres) may be covered with sections of **myelin** (myelinated fibre) separated by **nodes of Ranvier**. Thus involved in **saltatory conduction**.
- **Information** is chemically transmitted across a **synapse** by a **neurotransmitter**, which is released by a **presynaptic neuron** and **combines** with **receptors** on a **post synaptic neuron**.
- CNS also contains **glial cells**, which **sustain** the **neurons metabolically,** form **myelin (Oligodendrocytes**), and serve **as guides** for the neurons during **development**.
- The **brain** is **divided** into **six regions**: **Cerebrum, diencephalon, midbrain, pons, medulla** and **cerebellum**.
- The midbrain, pons and medulla form **brainstem** which contains **reticular formation** in its **central core** region.

- The **cerebellum** plays role in regulating **tone, posture, equilibrium, locomotion** and some kind of **memory** and programming.
- The cerebral **hemispheres** together with **diencephalon** form forebrain. The cortex is divided into **parietal, frontal, occipital** and **temporal lobes**.
- **Diencephalon** consists of **thalamus** and **hypothalamus**.
- The **limbic system** is a set of **deep forebrain structures** (like amygdala, hippocampus, fornix, cingulate gyrus, enterorhinal areas) associated with **emotions, learning, memory** and **discriminated behaviours**.
- The peripheral nervous system consists of **43 paired** nerves: **12 pairs** of **cranial**, **31 pairs** of **spinal**. Most nerves contain axons of afferent and efferent neurons.
- The effector division of the **PNS** is divided into **somatic** and **autonomic parts**, the somatic fibres **innervate muscles** and release transmitter **Ach**.
- The **autonomic part** innervates, **cardiac, smooth muscles, glands and GIT.**
- Each autonomic pathway consists of **preganglionic** neuron with its cell body in **CNS** and a **post ganglionic** neuron with its cell body in **autonomic ganglia** outside CNS.
- **Autonomic** preganglionic transmitter is **Ach** and post ganglionic sympathetic is **nor-epinephrine** and parasympathetic is again **Ach**.
- **Receptors** of parasympathetic transmission are **Nicotinic** (pre-ganglionic and neuromuscular junction) and **muscarinic** (post ganglionic).
- There are **alpha** and **beta adrenergic** receptors for **post ganglionic sympathetic fibres.**
- **Regeneration** occurs in **PNS** but **damaged neurons** in **CNS do not regenerate** or restore function.
- **Brain** tissue depends on a **continuous supply of glucose** and oxygen for metabolism.

- The **chemical** composition of **extracellular fluid** of the **CNS** is closely **regulated** by the **blood-brain barrier**.
- The **brain ventricles** (lateral, 3rd and 4th) and the space within meninges **(subarachnoid)** are filled with **cerebrospinal fluid**, which is formed by the **choroid plexus**.
- The resting membrane potential is due mainly to the diffusion of ions and determined by; the membrane's relative **permeability** to ions and **ionic** concentration **difference** across the membrane.
- Plasma membrane **Na^+, K^+ ATPase pump**, maintains intracellular **Na+ low** and **K^+ high**.
- In almost all resting membranes, plasma membrane is much more **permeable** to **K^+** than Na^+ and so the membrane potential is close to **Potassium equilibrium potential i.e,** inside **negative** relative to **outside**.
- **Two types** of cells are present in **CNS** (a) **Neurons** having no power of regeneration on injury (b) **connective tissue** cells, called neuroglia.
- The **neuroglia** is divided into **micro** and **macro-glial** cells.
- Microglia are **small dendritic cells**, increase in number by proliferation and are **scavengers** (phagocytic) in CNS.
- **Macroglia** include **astrocytes**, **oligodendro-cytes, Muller's cells** of retina, **Bergmann** glia of cerebellum, **pituitocytes** of neurohypophysis, **ependymal** and **choroidal** cells of ventricles and **satellite cells** of dorsal root and cranial nerve ganglia.
- Of these **astrocytes** are responsible for effective **blood brain and blood CSF barrier, oligo-dendrocytes** form **myclin** sheath and satellite cells encapsulate ganglia regulating their micro-environment.

- Glial cells **precursors** are present in the **adult brain** which on **multiplication** irrationally lead to development of **brain tumours.**

b. Cerebrospinal Fluid (CSF)

- CSF is present in the **ventricular system** of the **brain, subarachnoid** space of the brain and **spinal cord** and the central canal of spinal cord.
- CSF is **formed** mainly in the **choroid plexus** of the **lateral ventricles**, though ependyma and choroid plexuses of 3rd and 4th ventricles also contribute.
- CSF is formed by **active mechanism** and **ultra-filtration.**
- Rate of formation is **about 0.2–3 ml/min**, total amount is **150 ml** and pH is 7.3. Pressure is 100-200 mm H_2O.
- Content of **glucose, protein and K^+** is **lower** in CSF as compared to **plasma**, besides it contains lymphocytes 5/ml.
- CSF formed in **lateral ventricles** flows to **third** ventricle (foramen of Monroe), then to **fourth** ventricle (aqueduct of sylvius), then side tracked to **subarachnoid** space (foramen of Luschka and foramen of Magandie) but continue flowing through central canal of spinal cord.
- **Drainage** of CSF occurs **80%** through **dural sinuses** and **20% through spinal** veins.
- Main functions of CSF are: acts as **lymph** of the brain, provides proper chemical environment for neurons, **forms protective cushions** to brain, maintains constant internal volume of cranium (Monroe-Kelly doctrine), provides **nutrition** and **drains waste products** of nerve cells and is useful for diagnosing brain disorders as its composition reflects normal brain functioning.
- **Hydrocephalus** means **accumulation** of CSF in the cranium due to its **excessive** formation or **less** absorption.

- Lumbar puncture–a puncture done through introduction of needle into arachnoid space through intervertebral space between L_3 and L_4 and CSF is collected.
- The **puncture** is done to **analyse** CSF for **diagnosis** or to drain it to **relieve** pressure (as in hydrocephalus).
- **Caudal** anaesthesia is done to make **labor painless** (painless delivery particularly 1st and 2nd stage) and also for **ano-rectal** surgery. In this, anaesthesia is given in sacral canal through sacral hiatus.
- **Blood brain barrier** (BBB), is present between **blood** and the **interstitial fluid** of brain, supported by **astrocytes**. The expanded foot processes of astrocytes incompletely envelope the capillaries.
- Blood CSF barrier, the capillaries of choroid plexus show **gaps** between the **endothelial cells** of the capillary but the choroid epithelial cells that separate them from the CSF are joined by tight junctions.
- Functions of BBB include, **maintenance** of constant **chemical environment** around neurons (as fluctuations in K^+, Ca^{++}, Mg^{++} and H^+ can alter neuronal activity), **protects** brain from **endogenous** or **exogenous toxins** in the blood and **prevent** the escape of **neurotransmitters** into general circulation.
- CO_2, H_2O and O_2 **penetrate** through BBB easily, lipid soluble substance like **steroids** also pass through easily.
- **Proteins** or **protein bound** substances **do not** pass through BBB.
- H^+ and HCO_3^- and glucose can penetrate **slowly** through BBB.
- **Drugs** like **penicillin, chlor-tetracycline** enter the brain **slowly** but **sulpha drugs** and **erythromycin, L-DOPA** enter the brain **easily, dopamine does not** pass the **barrier.**

- **Circumventricular organs** are those structures of the brain which **donot** have **BBB**.
- These **organs** include, post pituitary, subfornical organ, organum vasculosum of lamina terminalis (OVLT), area postrema and median eminence.
- These organs are located **around** the **3rd ventricle** and are called **windows** of the **brain** as capillaries in these organs are fenestrated and are **highly permeable**.

c. Receptors, Receptor Potential and Action Potentials

- **Receptors** translate information from the external world (exteroceptors) and internal environment **(proprio and enteroceptors)** into **graded potential** which then generate **action potential**.
- Receptors may be either **specialized** ending of **afferent** neurons or separate cells adjacent to the neurons.
- Receptors respond best to **one form** of stimulus **energy** but they may respond to other energy forms if the stimulus intensity is **abnormally high.**
- **Activation** of receptor leads to perception of **one sensation** (the doctrine of specific nerve energy).
- **Application** of a **stimulus** to a **receptor**, opens **ions channels** in the receptor membrane. Ions then **flow across,** causing a **receptor potential.**
- Receptor potential **magnitude** and action potential **frequency** increases as stimulus strength **increases.**
- Receptor potentials can be **summated.**
- Neurons signal information by first **graded potentials** and then finally by **action potentials**.
- Graded potentials are **local potentials** that **die out** within 1-2 mm of their site of origin.
- Action potential (AP) is a **rapid change** in the membrane potential that occurs when **potential reverses** and membrane becomes **positive inside** (depolarized).

- AP occurs in **excitable membranes** because these contain **voltage-sensitive sodium channels,** which open as membrane depolarises, causing a positive feedback towards **sodium equilibrium potential**.
- AP **ends** as **Na^+ channels** close and K^+ channels **open**, restoring membrane potential.
- Depolarization of excitable membrane **triggers AP** only when membrane potential reaches **threshold**.
- Regardless of the **size** of **stimulus,** if the membrane reaches threshold the APs generated are all of the **same size**.
- A membrane is **refractory** for a **brief time** even though stimuli that were **previously effective** are applied.
- In a **myelinated fibre,** APs manifest **saltatory conduction.**
- APs can be initiated by receptors at the ends of afferent neurons, by synapses or in same cell by pacemaker potential.

d. Synapse

- **Synapse** is a **junctional** communication between **two neurons** having **physiological continuity** but not **anatomical union**.
- There are three types of synapses: (a) chemical (b) electrical and (c) conjoint.
- **Chemical** synapse involves a release of chemical **messanger** (neuro-transmitter). This type is present in all vertebrates including humans.
- **Electrical synapse**–in this transmission of impulses takes place by the transfer of **ions** directly, usually seen in **invertebrates**.
- **Conjoint** are the synapses where transmission is both chemical and electrical.
- **Interaction** of neurotransmitter with **receptor** at synapse leads to (a) activation of membrane **ion channels** (b) activation of **second messanger** system or (c) both.

- Second messanger system comprising G proteins when activated lends to (a) opening of ionic channels (through post synaptic neuron) (b) formation of cycle AMP or GMP (c) activation of intracellular enzymes directly by G proteins (d) activation of gene transcription leading to protein synthesis.
- Sequence of **events** at **presynaptic** membrane during synaptic transmission are (a) AP conducted to presynaptic terminal (b) depolarisation of presynaptic terminal (c) Ca^{++} channels open and Ca^{++} enters presynaptic terminal (e) vesicles fuse (docking) with the presynaptic membrane (f) rupture of vesicles and release of neurotransmitter.
- Sequence at post synaptic level–
  a. Neurotransmitter combines with receptors at sub synaptic membrane.
  b. This leads to either opening of **ligand** gated Na^{+} channels or opening of Ca^{++} channels or closure of K^{+} channels.
  c. Local **EPSP** develops.
  d. EPSPs at **soma-dendritic** tree are **integrated** at the **axon hillock** to develop **generator** and **action potential.**
  e. This is conducted in both directions, i.e. towards soma-dendritic tree and along the axon to the post synaptic neuron.
- Many **factors** like **toxins** (tetanus, botulinum), **pH, anoxia, anaesthetic** agents, **drugs** like caffeine, nicotine and benzidine, affect synaptic transmission.

e. Sensory Receptors

Two types of sensory receptors are:

a. **Exteroceptors**–Which collect information about the changes in the **outside** (extero) **environment** like telereceptors which are sensitive to smell, audition, vision (special senses) and exteroceptors like receptors for touch, pain, cold, warmth, pressure, tickle and itch, present on skin.

b. **Interoreceptors** which are sensitive to changes **inside** the body—hence adjudge the changes in **internal environment.**
   They can be:
   i. Visceral receptors (baro, chemo, osmo or pain) or
   ii. Proprioceptors (muscle spindle, golgi tendon organ, joint receptors like Pacinian and Ruffini and vestibular apparatus receptors.

f. Sensory System

- A single **afferent** neuron with all its **receptor** endings is a **sensory unit**.
- The **area** of body that, when **stimulated,** causes activity in a **sensory unit** or **other neuron** in the afferent pathway is called the **receptor field** of that neuron.
- The **specific** ascending pathways convey **information** about only a **single** type of information to sensory cortex.
- **Nonspecific** ascending pathways (ascending reticular system) conveys information from more than one type of **sensory unit** to the brainstem **reticular** formation and regions of **thalamus** not part of the specific ascending pathways.
- **Ascending** reticular activating system thus receives **collaterals** from specific ascending pathways and is responsible for **arousal** of **cortex**.
- **Three** relay stations on **sensory pathways** form essential circuitry for perception of any **sensation** i.e, 1st station **dorsal horn**, second **thalamus** and third **sensory** cortex.
- Stimulus **intensity** is **coded** by the **rate** of firing of **individual sensory units** and by the **number** of sensory units **activated**.

- **Location** of stimulus **depends** on the **size** of the **receptive field** covered by a single sensory unit and on the **overlap** of nearby **receptive** fields.
- Information coming into nervous system is **subject** to **control** by **ascending** and **descending** pathways.
- **Lateral inhibition** is a means by which ascending pathways **emphasise wanted** information and increase the **precision** of location of the stimulus.
- Information about **somatic sensation** enters both **specific** and non specific ascending pathways. The specific pathway **crosses** to the opposite side of the brain.
- The somatic sensations include **touch, pressure, proprioception** and **kinesthesia , temperature** and **pain**.
- The major receptor type responsible for **proprioception** and **kinesthesia** is the **muscle-spindle** stretch receptor.
- **Specific** receptors give rise to sensation of **pain**, which may induce **emotional** and **reflex** responses as well as **pain perception**.
- Stimulation produced **analgesia** and **TENS** control pain by blocking **pain pathways**.
- The sensations carried by **dorsal column** tracts are; **conscious proprioception** (joint movement and position), **unconscious extero** and **proprioception, vibration sense**, **fine touch**, **stereognosis**, **two point localisation** and **discrimination**.
- In conditions like **tabes dorsalis**, these sensations are gone and patient suffers from **'sensory ataxia'**.
- **Lateral spinothalamic** tract carries **pain** and **temperature** (contralateral side) and **anterior spinothalamic** tract carries **crude touch**, **pressure, sexual sensation, bladder sensation itching** and **tickle.**
- **Pain** producing **substances** are: bradykinin, K+, 5HT, Ach, AMP, substance P, histamine and PGE_2.

- Areas of brain for **pain localisation** is **somatosensory areas** 3, 1, 2 for **feeling** of pain it is **prefrontal lobe** whereas **pain perception** occurs in **thalamus** (dorso medial and intra laminar nucleus).
- Main **functions** of thalamus include:
  a. **Relay station** for specific sensations (vibration, pressure, stereognosis, conscious proprioception and sexual sensations).
  b. Perception for **crude sensation** (touch, pain).
  c. Relay station for **auditory** and **visual** sensation.
  d. **Control** for **smooth, slow** and **coordinated movements** (through its connection with basal ganglia, cerebellum and motor cortex).
  e. Role in short term **memory** and **emotions.**
  f. **Sleep wakeful** cycle (non specific ascending, diffuse reticular projection to cortex).

g. Spinal Organization of Movement

- **Movement** and **posture** depend on **coordinated contraction** of muscles operating around joints.
- Muscle **activity** depends on **discharges** of motor neurons innervating agonist muscles and causing their **contraction** and relaxation of **antagonists.**
- **Motor** systems in CNS coordinate muscle actions through control of motor neuronal activity in the **spinal cord.**
- Spinal motor neuron activity **(discharges)** also depends on many **spinal reflexes.**
- These **reflexes** are activated by **receptors** present in and around the muscles.
- **Activation** of **sensory receptors** then excites **interneurons** and motor neurons in the spinal cord and this **excitation triggers contraction** or **relaxation** of particular muscles.
- Most of the **descending projections** influence the activity of **interneurons** that are interposed

in **reflex circuits** and thus alter ongoing **spinal reflex activity.**

- In humans an **abrupt transaction** of the **spinal** cord results initially in a condition called **spinal shock**.
- Spinal shock is characterised by a **flaccid paralysis**, complete **areflexia, loss** of **autonomic function** and loss of all **sensation below** the level of the **transaction.**
- Spinal shock generally lasts for **3-4 weeks. Lower animals** have **less duration** of spinal shock (i.e. **frogs** a few **mins**, cats and **dogs** a few **days**).
- After spinal shock, **recovery starts,** first **flexor reflexes** return followed by **extensors,** hence terms **paraplegia** in **flexion** or **extension.**
- Thereafter reflexes become **hyperactive,** but **voluntary** movements and **sensations never return,** the paralysis changes character from flacidity to spasticity.
- The autonomic functions **return** but in **altered form** (i.e. bowel and bladder functions).
- **Hyperactivity** affects both the **muscle stretch reflexes** and **flexor reflexes.**
- Hyperactive stretch reflexes are associated not only with an increased resistance to **passive stretch** but also often with **clonus** (alternate contraction of agonists and antagonists) around joints such as ankle.
- Hyperactive flexion reflexes in response to **pain** stimulus applied to a foot, may include not only flexion of one or both lower extremities but also **urination**, **defication** and **sweating**.
- In **animals** spinal **transaction** produces **similar** changes but with **less period** of **shock,** therefore **spinal reflexes** can be **studied** in absence of **descending influences.**
- **Mid collicular** cut in midbrain, in animal results in **decerebrate rigidity** due to change in **balance** of excitatory and inhibitory motor control systems.

- As a result, some spinal reflexes such as the **flexion reflexes** are **suppressed** whereas others, such as **stretch reflexes** are **exaggerated**.
- **Muscle spindles** are complex **sensory receptors** (intrafusal fibres) lying parallel to regular (extra fusal) muscle fibers.
- Each spindle contains some **nuclear bag** and **chain fibres**. The former respond to **dynamic stretch** (rate of change of length of muscle fibre) and the latter to **adynamic sustained stretch**.
- **Ia** afferent fibres form **primary endings** on **nuclear bag** and chain fibres whereas **type II** afferent fibres form **secondary endings** on **nuclear chain fibres.**
- Dynamic γ ($\gamma1$) motor neurons end on **nuclear bag** fibres and static γ ($\gamma2$) motor neurons on **nuclear chain** fibres.
- Primary endings demonstrate both **static and dynamic** responses, which signal muscle **length** and **rate of change** in muscle length.
- **Secondary endings** demonstrate only **static response** and signal only **muscle length**.
- Gamma motor neurons cause muscle spindle to **shorten**, which prevent the unloading effect of muscle contraction.
- **Group Ib** afferents supply **golgi tendon** organs present in **series** in muscle tendon and respond to muscle contraction and loading (stretch)
- The stretch reflex includes (a) monosynaptic excitatory pathway from group Ia and type II muscle spindle afferents to α motor neurons (b) a **disynaptic inhibitory** pathway to antagonistic motor neurons.
- **Phasic** stretch reflexes are triggered by the **dynamic** responses of **group Ia** fibres and **tonic** stretch reflexes are triggered by the static responses of **type II** fibres.
- **Tapping** of muscle **Tendon** (knee or ankle jerk) will produce **burst** of electrical impulses in $\mathbf{I_A}$

afferent (primary afferent) fibres of the muscle spindle.

- Stimulation of **static gamma (γ_2)** to muscle spindle will cause increased **tonic stretch** reflex.
- Stimulation of **golgi tendon** organ in muscle causes inverse stretch reflex or **lengthening reaction**.
- Nociceptor stimulation results in polysynaptic flexor withdrawal reflex (mostly protective in nature).
- The **inverse** stretch reflex is elicited by **Ib afferents** of **golgi tendon** organs which **disynaptically** inhibit motor neurons of agonist muscles (**lengthening reaction**).
- **Flexor** reflexes are **polysynaptic** elicited by various receptors on the skin including **nociceptors**. These reflexes **excite flexor** group of muscles and **inhibit extensors.** The **opposite** pattern may occur **contralaterally**.
- The flexor **withdrawal** reflex is another more powerful form of flexor reflex elicited by **nociceptive** stimulation. It is protective in nature but has postural **crossed extensor component.**
- **Spinal reflexes** can be **experimentally** studied by **electrical** stimulation of the **afferect** fibres in nerves and recording **volleys** in the α **motor** axons from ventral root.
- **Principles** of reflex organisation derived from such studied include **spatial** and **temporal summation, occlusion** and various **patterns of inhibition.**

h. Descending Motor Systems

- Spinal **motor** neurons (lower motor neurons in **ventral grey**) are organised in a functional **topographic** manner.
- Motor neurons in the **lateral** ventral horn **innervate distal group** of **muscles** (Limb muscles) while those in **medial** ventral horn innervate **proximal** (axial or girdle) muscle.

- Similarly **lateral** and **medial** groups of **interneurons** synapse on the respective **lateral** and **medial** ventral **horn motor neurons.**
- Descending motor pathways can be divided into:
  a. **Lateral** system, which end on lateral **ventral horn** motor neurons directly or through corresponding **interneurons** to influence activity of **distal** group of muscles.
  b. **Medial** system, which ends on the medial group of **interneurons** and medial **ventral** horn neurons to influence **proximal** group of muscles.
- The lateral descending system includes the **lateral corticospinal** tract, and part of **corticobulbar tract** influencing distal musculature.
- The lateral system is involved in **fine**, **coordinated skilled** movements of the **limbs, digits, lower face** and **tongue.**
- The **medial** system includes the **ventral corticospinal, lateral and medial vestibulospinal, pontine** and **medullary reticulospinal** and **tectospinal tracts.**
- The medial system is involved in **controlling, tone, posture** and **manipulatory** movements in the **proximal** (axial or girdle muscles).
- Damage to the lateral system would result in **paucity** of fine **skillful** movements at the **distal joints.** Hence pure lateral corticospinal tract lesion will produce, **hypotonia**, **loss of skillful** and **fine movements** at the **periphery**.
- **Damage** to medial system would result in **tone** and **postural deficits** and deficits of **locomotion.**
- The medial system pathways which **originate** in the brainstem thus influence **tone**, **posture**, **locomotion** and **eye movements**.
- **Postural** reflexes include, **stretch reflex** (simplest), **crossed extensor reflex, several vestibular reflexes** (activation of extensors as a result of head movements, vestibulo-ocular reflex, vetibular placing reaction and ocular counter

rolling), the **tonic neck reflexes** and **righting reflexes.**

- Descending **monoaminergic** pathways affect the general level of **excitability** of spinal cord reflex circuits and ascending pathways.
- **Common** cause of motor disorder in humans is interruption of the **corticospinal tract** in internal **capsule resulting** in **capsular strokes**.
- The **resultant** disorder is often termed as **pyramidal tract syndrome** or **upper motor neuron disease**.
- **Characteristic** features of this disorder are:
  a. **Increased phasic** and **tonic** stretch **reflexes (Spasticity)** as there is also involvement of **extrapyramidal tracts**.
  b. Weakness of **distal group** of muscles.
  c. **Pathological** (altered) **reflexes** including **Babinski's signs.** (dorsiflexion of the big toe and fanning of other toes on stroking the sole of the foot).
  d. A **reduction** in **superficial reflexes** such as **abdominal, cremasteric.**
- If **only** the **corticospinal** tract is interrupted at the **medullary pyramid**, most of these signs **are absent**. There is distinct weakness of **distal muscles**, **paucity** of **skilled movement** and **positive Babinski's sign,** no spasticity rather **flaccidity** is seen.
- The corticospinal tract is named as **pyramidal tract** because on its way, in **medulla** it forms **pyramids**.

i. Motor Control—Cerebellum, Basal Ganglia

- Voluntary **movements** depend on **interactions** among motor areas of the **cerebral cortex, cerebellum** and **basal ganglia.**
- Cerebral **motor areas** include:
  a. **Primary** motor area (area 4) which forms origin of the **lateral motor system**, thus

controlling movements at distal group of muscles.

b. **Premotor area**, forming origin of the **medial system,** thus controlling proximal group of muscles.

c. **Supplementary** motor area, concerned with **planning** of **movement** along with **striatum.**

d. The frontal **eye fields** which help initiate **saccadic eye** movements.

- Cortical **motor** areas receive **sensory** inputs from **post central gyrus** (somatosensory area) and posterior parietal lobe, this feedback helps correct **motor commands**.
- The **cerebellum** influences the **rate, range, force** and **direction (synergy)** of movements. It also controls **muscle tone** and **posture** as well as **eye movements,** and **balance.**
- **To and fro** connection of **cerebellum** with **vestibular** and **reticular nuclei,** controls the **balance** and eye **movements**.
- The **spinocerebellum** receives inputs from **spinal cord** and **controls** the **proximal** group of **muscles** (tone, posture, equilibrium and progression) through its connections with tracts of **medial system** (cerebello-reticular, vestibular and rubral tracts).
- The **neocerebellum** receives **inputs** from motor **cortex** through **coricoponto cerebellar tracts** and influence **lateral system** and **distal group of muscles**.
- Most of the **inputs** to cerebellum is through pathways that end as **mossy fibres,** which evoke single action potential (simple spike) in **Purkinje cells.**
- The **inferior olive** projections to cerebellum end as **climbing fibres** which produce **repetitive discharges** of a **Purkinje cell**.
- **Complex spikes** are thought to alter the effectiveness of simple spikes and play a role in **motor learning**.

- The **output** of the **Purkinje cells** of cerebellum is **inhibitory** to the deep cerebellar **nuclei**.
- The **basal ganglia** include structures like **caudate, putamen, globus pallidus, substantia nigra** and **subthalamic** nucleus. They **interact** with **cerebral cortex**, and **thalamus**.
- The **input** from the subthalamic nucleus to the globus pallidus is **excitatory**.
- **Activity** transmitted from the cortex through basal ganglia can either **facilitate** or **inhibit** thalamic neurons that project to **motor cortex**.
- Thus basal ganglia affect the **output** of motor **cortex** (links medial and lateral system at cortical areas).
- Diseases of **cerebellum** and **basal ganglia** affect **motor** behaviour profoundly, the deficits caused by their lesions, can be understood on the basis of the interconnection of **cerebellum** and **basal ganglia** with **lateral** and **medial motor** system.
- Hence **Parkinson's** disease in **characterised** by, **rigidity** in proximal group of muscles, **flexion posture**, **short shuffling gait** (symptoms pertaining to medial system) and **resting tremor, pill rolling movements** (pertaining to lateral system).

j. CNS Motor Mechanism: Overview

- The **motor** nervous system comprises **motor cortex**, **basal ganglia**, **cerebellum** certain brainstem structures (vestibular nucleus, reticular nucleus, red nucleus, olivary nucleus), **descending** motor tracts (pyramidal and extrapyramidal) and **final common pathway** in the spinal cord (motor neurons of ventral grey).
- **Initiation** of motor activity is the function of cortical **association** areas.
- Basal ganglia and **lateral cerebellum** are concerned with planning, programming and coordination of voluntary movements.

- **Lateral** descending system (lateral corticospinal or pyramidal tract) is concerned with **execution** of **fine, skilled** movements at **periphery**.
- **Medial** descending system (extra pyramidal tracts) are concerned with **tone, posture, equilibrium** in **proximal** group of **muscles.**
- **Upper** motor neurons are the motor neurons above **the LMN**, present in the **brainstem**, **reticular formation, cerebral cortex** and **cerebellum**. Clinically UMN refers to **pyramidal** and **extrapyramidal tracts.**
- **Lower** motor neuron is the neuron present in the **anterior grey** horn and its equivalent for cranial nerve, located in their respective motor nuclei.
- **LMN** thus forms the **final common pathway** of motor output to different groups of muscles for the purpose of **movement.**
- The features of UMN **lesion** (pyramidal and extra pyramidal together) include, **contralateral spasticity**, **impairment of voluntary, skilled movements, exaggerated tendon** reflexes and **clonus**, Babinski's **positive** sign and **loss of superficial reflexes**.
- **Drugs** used for treatment of **Parkinson's disease** include, **L-DOPA, anticholinergic drugs** (atropine), **L-deprenyl** (MAO inhibitor) and **dopamine agonists** like **Bromocryptine.**
- Surgical **intervention** for Parkinson's disease include, **ablation** of motor **cortex**, sectioning of **cerebral peduncles** or **corticospinal** pathway, **destruction** of **medial** part of **globus pallidus**, section of **ansa lenticulars** and **destruction** of **ventro-lateral** nucleus of **thalamus.**
- **Implantation** of **foetal** brain nerve cells and adrenal **medullary** tissue near caudate may help in ameliorating the symptoms of Parkinson's disease.
- **Cerebellar** lesion is clinically **characterised** by:

  a. Charcots' triad (SIN: scanning speech, intention tremor, nystagmus).

b. LPR's tetrad (DDDD: dysmetria, decomposition, drunkan gait and dysdiadochokinesis).
c. Lucianis triad (AAA: asthenia, atonia and ataxia).

- Normal **gait** or walking is a pattern generated in the cervical and lumbar regions, coordinated by descending motor influences.
- Hence **abnormal gait** can be due to:
  a. Motor deficiency.
  b. Lack of proper feedback.
  c. Structural malformation of locomotor apparatus.
- Some abnormal **gaits** are:
  1. **Spastic gait**–seen in hemiplegia (lesion in internal capsule), patient walks on a narrow base, with extended lower limbs, brings **limb** inward in an arc, the toes scrapping along the floor.
  2. **Drunkan gait**–as in cerebellar ataxia, patient fails to walk on a straight line, deviating sidewards with zigzag walking.
  3. **Festinant gait**–as in Parkinsonism, short shuffling gait with flexed trunk, as if patient catching the centre of gravity by brisk, automatic walking.
  4. **Stamping gait** as in sensory ataxia of tabes dorsalis, patient raises foot suddenly and brings it to the ground with a stamp.
  5. **High stepping gait** seen in common peroneal nerve palsy the limbs are raised to higher level to avoid tripping from the toes catching the ground.
  6. Waddling gait seen in myopathies and muscular dystrophies affecting the truncal, pelvic and thigh muscles, body shows lumbar lordosis and feet are placed widely apart.
- **Features** of LMN **lesion** include; damage to anterior horn cell, **flaccid paralysis, deep reflexes** are **lost** or hypoactive, **atrophy** of paralysed **muscles, atonia,** no voluntary movement,

EMG shows **fibrillation** and **fasciculation potentials,** electrical responses abnormal–usually seen in **poliomyelitis** and **motor neuron disease (MND).**

- **Lesion** of **ventromedial** (VM) nucleus of hypothalamus (so called satiety area) causes **hyperphagia** and **obesity.**
- Since VMN inhibits the activity of LH (feeding centre) it decides the food intake. **VMN** is also called **glucostat.**
- The **activity** of **VMN** (glucostal) depends on A–V glucose difference or blood glucose level.
- Hence **hyperglycemia** stimulates VMN, which **inhibits** LH and food intake and **hypoglycemia** causes **opposite effect** i.e. **increase** in **food intake.**
- **Thirst centre** in hypothalamus is stimulated by:
  a. Increased osmolarity of ECF.
  b. **Decrease** in ECF **volume** (through **baroreceptors, angiotensin II** acting on **subfornical** organ).
  c. Factors like **dryness** of mouth (oral and pharyngeal mucosa).
  d. **Psychological** factors.
- Functions of **hypothalamus** include:
  a. Regulation of **food intake.**
  b. **Temperature** regulation.
  c. Regulation of **thirst.**
  d. Regulation of **ECF volume.**
  e. Regulation of **endocrines** (ant and post pituitary).
  f. Controls **reproduction.**
  g. Reproductive **behaviour.**
  h. **Sleep wakeful** cycle.
  i. Centre of **autonomic** function (head ganglion).
  j. **Emotions.**
  k. Biological **rhythms.**
  l. **Reward** and **punishment.**
  m. **Somato-visceral** integration.

- **Reticular formation** consists of diffuse **network** of **nerve fibres, scattered, ill defined, phylogenetically very old**, mostly lying in the **core** of the **brainstem extending** from upper part of **cervical spinal cord** to **diencephalon**, in which are **scattered** many **cell-sized** nonspecific **neurons.**
- **Functions** of **reticular formation,** include: control of **muscle tone** (through reticulospinal tracts), **sleep** and **wakefulness** (through ARAS), influence **autonomic** and **visceral functions** (through vital centres located in reticular formation like vasomotor, respiratory, CTZ), **influence EEG** (through ARAS), process of **learning** and **memory** and **neuroendocrine** control (through hypothalamus).
- Ascending reticular activating system (ARAS) is concerned with generalised cortical **arousal** and its activity is influenced by many factors like, **collaterals** from **specific** ascending **sensory pathways**, cortical **activation** of ARAS, circulating **catecholamines, thyroid** hormones and **various drugs** acting on CNS (CNS depressants, anaesthetic agents, tranquilisers).
- Some important **sleep disorders** are:
  a. **Somnambulism** (sleep walking).
  b. **Sleep apnoea** (obstructive or central in nature).
  c. **Narcolepsy** (irresitible desire to sleep during working).
  d. **Nocturnal bed wetting** (nocturnal enuresis).
  e. **Sleeping sickness** (caused by T. Gambiens and T. cruzi).
  f. REM **behavioral** disorders.
- **Synchronisation** of EEG (shifting from faster β to slower α rhythm) is caused by **rhythmical** discharge of stimulation at a **low frequency** rate of some **sub cortical** areas, **rhythmical discharge** of impulses from **thalamus** and **synchronous** effect of adjacent neighbouring parallel fibres.
- Many **factors** influence **EEG** waves, these include:
  a. **Catecholamines** (produce β rhythm by acting on ARAS).

b. **Anaesthetic** agents (induce α or δ rhythm).
c. **Hypoglycaemia** (decrease in α rhythm).
d. **Hypothermia,** and
e. **Hypercapnia** (decrease α rhythm).

- Bitemporal lobe ablation in animal causes a syndrome known as Kluver Bucy syndrome, which is characterized by **visual agnosia** (inability to recognise), **oral tendencies**, abnormal **mounting** even on other species animals **(hypersexuality)**, **hypermetamorphosis** (peculiar attention of different objects), changes in **emotional** behaviour (no signs of fear), changes in **dietary** habits (monkeys usually vegetarian start accepting meat), **word deafness** and loss of **recent memory**.
- **Learning** is based on and studied by **conditioned reflexes** (reflex response is obtained on giving or pairing conditioned stimulus (CS) with unconditioned (UCS) stimulus. Two types of conditioned **reflexes**:
  a. **Classical** (Pavlovian conditioning), pairing of CS with UCS after sometimes only CS produces response.
  b. Instrumental i.e. escape or avoidance and operant conditioning. Responses to CS are either escape (foot shock) or reward (pressing a bar getting food pellet as reward).
- The term **aphasia** means inability to comprehend or produce or write language.
- Types of aphasia include:
  a. **Pure** word blindness or **deafness** (lesion in audio or visual psychic areas).
  b. **Wernicke's** aphasia (sensory or fluent aphasia).
  c. **Broca's** aphasia (non fluent motor aphasia).
  d. **Global aphasia** (lesion in wernick's and surrounding areas).
- Water **intake** is increased by the action of angiotensin II or receptors in the subfornical region of the brain.

Chapter Twelve

Special Senses

a. Chemical Senses (Smell and Taste)

- The chemical senses are **olfaction (sense of smell)** and **gustation (sense of taste).**
- The **olfactory receptors** are located in the **epithelium** below the **third turbinal** plate in the **nose.** The **receptor proteins** are located in the cilia of the **olfactory neurons.**
- These receptors are **multimodal** i.e. each receptor responds to **more** than one **odour.** So **specific odours** are coded in the **pattern** of **information** that reaches **brain.**
- In many **animals** through pheromones, olfactory stimuli play an **important role** in **sexual behaviours,** although this is not strikingly evident in humans.
- The **taste receptors** are found primarily on **tongue.**
- Taste sensations reach the **cerebral cortex** primarily via **facial** (VIII) and **glossopharyngeal** (IX) cranial nerves.
- The **facial nerve (chorda tympani)** supplies **anterior two thirds** of the **tongue** while the **glossopharyngeal** nerve innervates the **vallate papillae at the posterior one third** of the tongue.
- The taste buds on the **walls** of the mouth and **soft palate** are innervated by the **vagus (X) nerve.**
- These **nerves subserving taste**, project to the **nucleus of tractus solitarius (NTS)** in the medulla. From the NTS taste sensations project to the **thalamus** and the **lateral region** of the **post central gyrus** adjacent to somatic area for **tongue**.

- **Taste afferents** from NTS also play a role in various visceral reflexes. (i.e. secretion of **saliva, gastric juice).**
- The sense of taste is important in **discriminating** between **different foodstuffs** and in regulating some **gastrointestinal secretions.**
- The **stimulus** to which a receptor is most **sensitive** is called as **adequate** stimulus.
- When a receptor is **constantly** activated, the **rate** of discharge of its afferent fibre will tend to **fall** with time. This is known as **accommodation.**
- The initial step in sensory transduction varies with receptor type. There is then a change in the number of open ions channels, which results in generation of the **receptor** potential.
- The **frequency** of a train of action potentials in an afferent fibre **reflects** the **intensity** of the stimulus given to its receptor.
- The receptive **fields** of adjacent touch receptors **overlap**.
- Touch is subserved by a number of **different** types of **receptors** including bare nerve endings. The **size** of the receptor field of touch receptors varies, being **smallest** in the finger tips, lips, and tip of tongue and largest on the back.
- The **epicritic** (fine) touch from skin reaches the brain via the **dorsal** column **tracts** and nuclei.
- The **spinothalamic** tract relays information of **pain, crude touch** and **temperature**.
- Pain **receptors** are **free** nerve endings and they are activated by pain producing **chemicals** including **bradykinin**.
- **Fast** component of **pain** is transmitted through large diameter **Aδ** myelinated fibres whereas **slow** pain is transmitted through unmydinated **C fibres**.
- Pain arising from the **visceral** organs is **unpleasant** in quality **poorly** localised and may be **referred** to **skin** segments of similar dermatomal origin.

- The signals from the somatosensory systems (**Lemniscal** and **spinothalamic**) reach **consciousness** in the **post central gyrus** (Area 3,1,2), which does not appear to receive any signals from **nociceptors**. Hence pain cannot be elicited on stimulation of the primary sensory cortex.

b. Taste and Smell

- The receptors for taste **(taste buds)** are found throughout the mouth, principally on the **tongue** and can response to many different substances (sweet, sour, salt, bitter).
- Taste sensation from **anterior 2/3** of tongue is carried by **chorda tympani** (facial nerve) and **posterior 1/3** of tongue by **glossopharyngeal** nerve.
- Olfactory receptors are part of the afferent olfactory **neurons**, lie in the mucosa in the **upper nasal cavity**.
- Odorant **molecules** once **dissolved** in the **mucus** that bathes the olfactory receptors are transported to the **receptors** by odorant binding **proteins**.
- Olfactory **pathways** go the **limbic system**.
- All sensory information going to primary sensory cortex is elaborated after it is relayed to a cortical **association area**.
- Regions of **association** area are near to **sensory area**.
- **Bitter** taste sensation is located in the taste buds of the **posterior third** of the tongue.
- Lesion of **seventh cranial** nerve results in **loss** of **taste** sensation from **anterior 2/3** of the tongue.
- Smell of **ammonia**, stimulates **sensory interneurons** of the **olfactory bulb**.
- Anterior olfactory nucleus, pre-piriform cortex and amygdala and entero-rhinal areas of brain are involved in sense of smell.

c. Vision

- The **intraocular pressure** is the result of the **balance** between the **secretion** and **drainage** of **aqueous humour**.
- The secretion is **active** and is **reduced by drugs** that **inhibit enzyme carbonic anhydrase.**
- The **diameter** of the **pupils** is controlled by **sympathetic innervation** from the **superior cervical ganglion** (muscle **dilator pupillae**) and by **parasympathetic nerves** from the **ciliary** ganglion (muscle **sphincter pupillae).**
- The **pressure** within the eye the **IO, (intraocular pressure)** is about **15 mmHg (2 kpa).**
- In **light reflex,** when light is shone in one eye, **both pupils constrict** (via centre of **Adinger westphal nucleus**). They also **constrict** when **eye** is focussed on **near object** (accommodation) three responses occur:
  a. **Constriction** of pupils.
  b. **Conjugate** derivation of the eyes.
  c. **Anterior surface** of the lens becomes more **convex** (diopteric power of the eye increases).
- In **Argyl Robertson Pupil** (ARP), accommodation reflex is present whereas **light reflex is gone** (Lesion pretectal region).
- The main **refractive element** of the eye is the **cornea.** The lens is the **focussing element.**
- Total refractory power of the **schematic eye** is **+ 59 diopters, Lens** contributes about **+ 16 diopters** and **cornea +43 diopters**.
- When the eye is **focussed on a near object** the ciliary **muscle contracts, relaxes the lens capsule, anterior surface of lens bulges** (becomes more convex). Ciliary muscle relaxes on focussing distant object.
- **Myopia (short sightedness), Hypermetropia** (long sighted) and **astigmatism** are the main **refractory errors** of the eye.

- In **myopia**, either the **lens** system of the eye is too strong (more dioptric **power > 59D)** or the **eye ball** is **too long**. The image of **distant object** is formed in **front of retina**—corrected by **biconcave lens.**
- In **hypermetropia,** either the lens system is **weak** (power < 59D) or eye ball is short, image of distant object in formed **behind the retina**—corrected by **biconvex lens.**
- **Fovea centralis** is **highly concentrated** with **cones** and periphery of retina (parafovial) **with rods.**
- Hence **visual acuity** is a **function of cones** in fovea. In good light, the visual acuity falls towards the edge of the visual field.
- **Full dark adaptation** takes about **30 mins** and during this period visual acuity is **best in the parafovial region** (where rods are very dense).
- The fovea has **no rods**, only **cones.**
- **Colour vision** requires **stimulation** of the **cones** which are active in **bright light (photopic vision)**.
- **Protanopes lack** the **pigment** for **detecting red light**.
- **Deuteranops, lack** the **pigment** for **detecting green light**.
- Hence **red and green color blinds** (Protanopes and deuteranopes) are **professional hazards** as **drivers, pilots**.
- Light is described by its **wavelength** or **frequency**.
- The **light** falling on **retina** must be focussed by the **cornea** and **lens.**
- Lens **curvature** and **shape** are changed in response to viewing **near** or **distant** objects, so that both are focussed on retina.
- **Presbyopia** interferes with **accommodation** (due to non-ability of lens to change its curvature to view **near objects**). Can be corrected by using **bifocal lens**.

- **Cataract** (opacity of lens) **prevents** the **passage** of light to the **retina.**
- An eyeball **too long** or **too short** relative to focussing power of the lens causes **short sightedness** (myopia) or **farsightedness** (hypermetropia).
- **Rods** and **Cones** are **visual receptors** in the retina. They consist of protein **opsin** and a **chromophore**.
- When light falls on chromophore, the **photic energy** causes the chromophore to **change shape**, which triggers a **cascade** of events involving the second **messanger** cyclic **GMP** and Ca^{++}.
- The cones are **sensitive** to **bright light (photopic)** and rods to dim light **(Scotopic)** or twilight (evenings and dawns).
- The **colours,** we perceive are related to the **wavelength** of light. Different wavelengths excite one of the **three cone** photopigment most strongly.
- Thus **colour** vision is a function of **cones.**
- The rods and cones **synapse** on **bipolar cells,** which synapse on **ganglion cells.**
- Ganglion cell **axons** form **optic nerves,** half of the optic nerve fibres **(nasal half** from each retina) **cross** to the opposite side of the brain in the **optic chiasm**.
- Fibres in the **optic tract** terminate in the **lateral geniculate body** of the thalamus, which send fibres to **visual cortex.**
- **Visual** information is also relayed to **brain areas.** (hypothalamus pineal). **Controlling** the **biological rhythms** of the body.
- **Coding** in the visual system occurs along **parallel pathways** in which different aspects of **visual information,** such as **colour, form, movement** and **depth** are kept separate from each other.
- **Near** point of **vision** is the nearest point to the eye at which an object can be brought into **focus** by **accommodation**. This point is **nearest** is

infancy and **childhood** and **recedes** throughout **life** but rapidly with **advancing age.**

- This **recession** is due principally to increasing **hardness** of the **lens**, with a resulting **loss of accommodation** due to the steady decrease in degree to which the **curvature** of lens can be increased.
- By the age of 40-45, the **loss** of accommodation is sufficient to making **reading** and **close work** difficult. This condition is known as **presbyopia** and can be corrected by wearing glasses with **convex lens** (reading glasses).
- **Near Response:** In addition to accommodation the **visual axes converge** and pupils **constrict** when an individual looks an a **near object**. This **three**-part response (a) **accommodation** (b) **convergence** of the visual axes (c) pupillary **constriction** is called the **near response.**
- Astigmatism is a condition in which the **curvature** of cornea is not uniform in all its meridians. The **image** formed is **blurred**. It is corrected by **cylindrical** lens placed in such a way that they **equalize refraction** in all meridians.
- Individuals with normal **colour vision** are called **trichromatic** they have all **three cone systems.**
- **Dichromates** are individuals with only **two cone** system—they may have protanopia, deuteranopia or tritanopia (term 'anopia' means color blind). Can **match** their color spectrum by using **two primary** colors.
- Monochromats have only **one cone** system can match their color by **varying** the **intensity** of only one primary color.
- **Visual threshold** is the **minimum** amount of light that **elicits** a sensation of light.
- **Visual acuity** is the **degree** to which the **details** and **contours** of objects are **perceived**.
- The **snellen charts** are designed so that the height of the letters in the smaller line, a normal individual can read at 20 ft **subtends** a visual angle of **5 minutes**. Each of the lines in the letters are

separated by **1 minute** of arc. Thus a minimal separable in a normal individual corresponds to a visual angle of 1 min.

- **Critical fusion frequency** is the **rate** at which visual **stimuli** can be **presented** and still be **perceived** as **separate** stimulis. Stimuli presented at a **higher rate** than **CFF** are perceived as **continuous** stimuli. **Motion** picture **frames** are presented above CFF and movie begins to flicker when projectors slow down.
- The **point** on the **retina** on which the images of an object must fall, if it is to be seen **binocularly** as a **single** object are called **corresponding points.**
- Diplopia (double images) results if images don't fall on corresponding points in the retina.
- **Field** of vision **defects** are referred to as **homonymous** anopia (same side of both visual fields), **hemianopia** (half field defect or half blindness).
- **Lesions** of **optic nerve** produce **blindness** in the eye.
- Lesion in **one optic tract** causes blindness is half of the visual field **(homonymous hemianopia)**
- Lesions affecting **optic chiasma** produce **heteronymous** hemianopia (since fibres from both nasal hemiretinas decussate).
- A **pituitary tumour** pressing upon **optic chiasma** causes loss of field of vision called bitemporal hemianopia.
- The **inferior temporal** region of the cerebral cortex is involved in **recognition of face.**

d. Hearing

- The **range of hearing** in human ear is **20 Hz—20 kHz**.
- The **ear** is **most sensitive** to **frequencies between 1 to 3 kHz.**
- The **ossicles** of the **middle ear** are essential for the **efficient transmission** of airborne sounds to the cochlea.

- The **endolymph** unlike **blood plasma**, is high in potassium and low in **sodium content**.
- In **conductive hearing loss,** bone conduction would be **near normal** while air conduction would be **impaired**.
- If the weber is **localised** to the **normal ear** it indicates **damage to the cochlear hair cells**.
- In Rinne test if **bone conduction** is **better** than **air condition** in one ear, it indicates otitis media of that ear.
- **Adequate** and **repeated click** stimulation of the **cochlea** illicits **series of potentials** along **auditory pathways,** which are **volume conducted** to the **vertex**. These potentials are known as **Brainstem auditory evoked potentials (BAEPs).**
- These potentials **(I-V)** indicate **functional integrity of pathways** in **brainstem. Site of lesion** in auditory pathways can be detected by BAEP.
- The **pitch** of the average **male voice** in conversion is about **120 Hz** and that of **female** voice about **250** Hzs.
- Pitch **discrimination** is best in the **1000 to 3000 Hz** range and is poor at high or low pitches.
- The tympanic membrane acts as a **resonator**, very nearly **critically damped**. The ossicles in the middle ear function as a **lever system** converting tympanic resonance into **movements** of **stapes**. This **increases** sound **pressure** that arrives at **oval winded** about **1 to 3 times.**
- **Sound** energy is transmitted by movement of pressure **waves**.
- Sound wave **frequency** determines **pitch**, and amplitude determine **loudness**.
  a. Sound waves enter the ear canal and press against the **tympanic membrane**, causing it to **vibrate**.
  b. The vibrating membrane causes movement of the **three middle ear ossicles** and the **stapes** presses against the **oval window** membrane.

c. Movements of this membrane set up pressure waves in the **fluid filled scala vestibuli**, which cause movements in the **cochlear duct wall,** setting up **pressure waves** in fluid there.
d. These pressure waves cause **vibrations** in the **basilar membrane**, located on one side of cochlear duct.
e. As the membrane vibrates the hair **cells** of the **organ of Corti move** in relation to the **tectorial membrane.**
f. **Movements** of the hair cells **stereocilia** stimulate them to release **neurotransmitter** that activates **receptors** on the peripheral ends of the **afferent nerve** fibre (cochlear nerve).

- Each **part** of the **basilar** membrane **vibrates** maximally in response to one particular sound **frequency (tonotopic localisation)**.

e. Vestibular Apparatus (System)

- Vestibular apparatus consists of **utricle , saccule** and **three semicircular** canals situated in the temporal bone on each side of the head, form vestibular component of inner ear.
- The ampulla in the **semi circular** canals detect **angular** acceleration/deceleration duration **rotation** of the head.
- The **otolith organs** are **gelatinous substances** present in **utricle** and **saccule** , their hair cells move in response to change in **linear acceleration** and the position of the head relative to **gravity**.
- The **direction** of **hair** in utricle is **horizontal** and that in saccule is **vertical.** Hence bending of **head forward** or backward (flexion or extension) will stimulate hair cells in utricle and bending head **on shoulder** will stimulate hair cells of **saccule**.
- **Vestibular apparatus** of the ear consists of:
  a. Utricle and saccule.
  b. Semi circular canals.

- The **otolith organs** in the ampulla of **utricle** and **saccule** respond to **pull of gravity.**
- As **direction of hairs is horizontal** in **saccule**, they get stimulated on **bending of head side-wards over shoulders.**
- These otolith organs **regulate posture** by initiating **vestibular postural reflexes,** to adjust position of body with change in **head position**.
- The **semicircular canals** and the **chambers of the utricle and saccule** contain **endolymph** as does the **scala media** of the **cochlea.**
- The semicircular canals are **stimulated** with **angular acceleration/deceleration** and are **important for control** of **eye movements**.
- When an **object is rotated** in a **swivelling chair**, the eyes tend to **fixate** on one object until the eyes reach the **limit of their movement**, whereupon they fixate on **another**. The alteration between **smooth pursuit movements and the** subsequent saccade is **optokinetic nystagmus**. If the eyes are defocused, however they cannot fixate and a vestibular nystagmus become evident.

Chapter Thirteen

Higher Brain Functions

a. Learning and Memory

- **Motivations** (rewards and punishments) are generally **crucial** to learning.
- Working memory has **limited** capacity, is **short term** and depends on functioning **brain electrical** activity.
- After registering in working memory, **facts** either **fade** away or are **consolidated** in **long term** memory, depending on **attention, motivation** and **various** hormones.
- Long term memory, of which there are two forms—**procedural** and **declarative** —seems to have an unlimited capacity and to be **independent** of brain electrical activity.
- Memory **traces** are localised, discrete brain areas containing **cellular** or **molecular** changes specific to discrete memories.
- Learning is **enhanced** after subjects are exposed to **enriched** environments. The enhancement is presumably due to the brain **neural** and **chemical** development that follows such **exposure.**
- In **90%** of the population, the **left hemispheric dominance** is seen for producing **language** and in performing other **tasks** that require rapid changes over time.
- After **damage** to the **dominant** hemisphere, some language function can be acquired by the **opposite** hemisphere, the **younger** the patient, more **greater** the tasks of function.

- Many brain **units** are involved in the performance of even simple mental **task.**
- Each unit is localised to a specific **brain area**, but because many units are involved, **widely distributed** brain areas take part in **mental tasks.**
- Natural **opioid** are **polypeptides**, released in different parts of the body and **modulate** physiological activities.
- **Enkephalins** and **endorphins** are the two types of natural opioids.
- Endorphins are further divided into (a) β–endorphin (b) Dynorphin and (c) Neo-endorphins.
- Main functions of endorphins are to **modulate synaptic transmission** in particular to influence **pain** mechanisms in brain stem, spinal cord and releasing hormones of hypothalamus-pituitary axis.
- Reflexes can be (a) **inborn** (unconditioned) and (b) **conditioned**. Unconditioned reflexes are the inborn or inherent reflexes e.g. secretion of saliva or gastric juice when food is placed in mouth.
- **Conditioned** reflexes are **acquired** ones e.g. salivation on thought of food or ringing of the bell (Pavlov's conditioning).
- Reflexes may be **asynaptic** (axon reflex), **mono-synaptic** (stretch reflex), **disynaptic** (inverse stretch reflex) and **polysynaptic** (withdrawal reflex).

b. Memory Speech, EEG

- **Learning** is **laying down** of a **store of knowledge** that can be used as a **guide to future activity**.
- It is a **complex process** that can be classified (a) Associative (b) non associative learning.
- All learning must involve **changes** in the **connections** between the **neurons** involved in **specific tasks**.
- **Memory** is the name given to this **laid down store** of knowledge. It is **not localised** but is

distributed through a number of **neural networks**, each of which is involved in **some task**.

- **Loss of memory** is called **amnesia**. Inability to **recall** events that occurred **before** an **incident** in **retrograde amnesia,** while inability to recall events that occurred **after an incident** is **antegrade amnesia**.
- The **speech centre** is located in the **left hemisphere** in most people including left handed. Frontal speech area (Brodman's No. 42) is known as **Broca's area**.
- The **frontal lobes** are involved in **motor control.**
- **Damage** to the parietal lobes can led to failure to **object recognition**.
- The **EEG** of a **normal awake** adult is dominated by **beta waves**.
- **During deep sleep** The EEG is dominated by **delta wave activity** but is **interrupted** by **beta-like** activity during **episodes of REM sleep**.
- **Since EEG** during **rapid eye movement sleep** is similar to that of **wakeful state** (dominated by **beta rhythm**), REM sleep is also known as **paradoxical sleep (paradox in EEG)**.
- The EEG can be used to monitor **health** of **brain**.
- The slowing or presence of slow EEG rhythm i.e., **delta waves** in awake person is **indicative** of **cerebral pathology**.
- During normal sleep, **secretion** of **cortisol** and some other hormones (growth hormone) is increased.
- **Recording** of **brain potentials** by **scalp electrodes** is **EEG**.
- **German psychiatrist Hans Berger analysed these potentials in a systematic fashion** and described them as EEG.
- **Characteristic** of **EEG** waves: Four waves.
  a. **Alpha rhythm:** Seen in **awake**, **mind** not **involved in arithmetical calculation** (mental rest), and **eyes closed, subject,** frequency 8 to 12 Hz/sec, amplitude 50-100 μv. Most marked in **parieto-occipital** area.

b. **Beta rhythm:** Seen over **frontal region**. Frequency of 18 to 30 Hz/sec, amp. very low. Dominant rhythm during **wakeful** and **alert stage**.

c. **Theta rhythm: 4 to 7 Hz/sec,** occurs in **children** and generated in **hippocampus**.

d. **Delta waves:** Frequency **0.5 to 4 Hz/sec,** seen in **deep sleep**.

- **Frequency of alpha** is **decreased** by **low blood glucose** level, a **low body temperature**, a low level of adrenocortical hormones and **high arterial PCO_2.**
- **Alpha block: When attention** is focussed on **something**, alpha is **replaced** by somewhat **irregular low voltage activity** this is called as **alpha block**.
- **Insomnia** may be defined as the **subjective problem** of **insufficient** or non restorative **sleep despite** an adequate **opportunity** for **sleep**, occurs at one time or another in **almost all adults**.
- **Narcolepsy** is a **disease** in which there is **episodic sudden loss** of **muscle** tone and an eventually irresistible urge to sleep **during day time** activities.
- **Sleep apnoea:** Episodes of apnoea (cessation of breathing) during sleep can be **central** in **origin**, i.e. due to failure of discharge in the nerves producing respiration or they can be due to airway obstruction (obstructive sleep apnoea).

c. Consciousness and Behaviour

- Consciousness includes, conscious **experiences** and **states** of consciousness. The **EEG** provides one means of defining the state of consciousness.
- Electric currents in the cerebral cortex due predominantly to **summed** postsynaptic potentials are recorded as the EEG.
- **Slower** EEG waves correlate with **less responsive behaviours.**

- Rhythm generators in the **thalamus** are probably responsible for the **wave like nature** of EEG (recruiting response of thalamus).
- **Alpha** rhythm and during EEG arousal, **beta** rhythm characterize EEG of a **awake** person.
- **Slow wave** sleep progresses from stage 1 (faster, lower amplitude waves) through stage 4 (slower, higher amplitude waves) followed by an **episode** of REM (paradoxical) sleep.
- There are generally **five** of these cycles **per night,** each cycle having **2/3 SWS** alternating with **1/3** REM).
- In the brainstem, a sleep producing system and an arousal system interact to produce **sleep-wake** cycles.
- Brain structures involved in directed attention, particularly the **locus ceruleus**, are thought to determine which area of the brain gain temporary predominance in the ongoing stream of conscious experience.
- Conscious experience depends on directed **attention**, which occurs due to activity in **interacting neuron** network.
- For such an experience to occur, **neural** activity **must** be present in the **brain** for a minimum period of time.
- Neural processes that result in perceptions, judgments, problem-solving ability, and discriminate responses to stimuli can occur even though conscious experience do not develop.

Chapter Fourteen

Autonomic Nervous System

- **Hypothalamus** is the **head ganglion** of autonomic nervous system. It **regulates** the **homeostatic activity of ANS**.
- **Sympathetic preganglionic** neurons are found in spinal segment from $\mathbf{T_1}$**-**$\mathbf{L_2}$**.**
- **Paired sympathetic ganglia** are found on **both sides** of **spinal cord** from the **cervical region** to the **sacral region**.
- In the cervical region, only **three pairs of ganglia** (superior, middle and inferior) are found while from T_1 to L_3, there **is a pair** of ganglia for each **spinal segment**.
- **Thoraco-lumbar outflow** (the lateral horn of spinal cord) from T_1-L_2 form the connector neurons of sympathetic system.
- **Sympathetic preganglionic** fibres secrete **acetyl choline as neurotransmitter** and post ganglionic produce **nor-epinephrine.**
- Although majority of blood vessels are innervated by **sympathetic vasoconstrictor fibres,** some, such as those in the **salivary glands, and exocrine pancreas**, also have a vasodilator **parasympathetic innervation.**
- **Parasympathetic** preganglionic fibres are found in **cranial nerves III, VII, IX and X.**
- The **salivary glands** are innervated by **parasympathetic vasodilator** fibres, which promote salivary secretion.
- **Both parasympathetic, pre** and **post ganglionic fibres** secrete **acetyl choline** as **neurotransmitter**.

- The **acetyl choline receptor** in both **parasympathetic** and **sympathetic ganglia** are **nicotinic** and can be blocked by **curare.**
- **Acetylcholine** secreted by **parasympathetic post ganglionic** fibres acts on **muscarinic** receptors which can be blocked by **atropine**.
- **Epinephrine** and **norepinephrine** are secreted by the **adrenal medulla** in response to stimulation of **sympathetic preganglionic** travelling in the splanchnic nerve.
- Stimulation of sympathetic nerves to the **eyes** results in **dilation** of the **pupils**.
- Although activation of sympathetic nerves causes **generalized vasoconstriction, epinephrine** secreted by adrenal **medulla** acts on **β-adrenoceptors** of the blood vessels of the **muscles** to **cause vasodilatation.**
- **Norepinephrine** acts preferentially **on α-adrenoceptors, epinephrine** acts on **β-adrenoceptors.** Ordinarily both these transmitters can act on α and β adrenoceptors.
- Stimulation of **parasympathetic** to eye, cause **pupillary constriction,** stimulation of **parasympathetic** to GIT (vagus) cause enhanced **motility of GI tract.**
- **Sympathetic** stimulation to **tracheo-bronchial** tree causes relaxation of smooth muscle hence **bronchodilation**.
- The **sacral outflow** of parasympathetic (S_2-S_4) supplies the pelvic viscera via the pelvic nerves.
- Finding out **variation** in systolic, diastolic BP and heart rate, on change of posture, deep breathing or isometric exercise, forms the **basis** for bed side **tests** for ANS.
- These tests are, **standing** test for orthostatic hypotension, **deep breaths** tests, **hand grip** test and **valsalva test.**
- The effect of stimulation of **post ganglionic** sympathetic fibres is mediated through α or β or both **adrenergic** receptors.

- **Stimulation** of α causes, vasoconstriction, contraction of sphincters, mydriasis (dilatation of pupil), pilomotor erection and decrease in insulin secretion.
- **Stimulation** of β **receptors** cause, increase in heart rate and force of contraction, lipolysis (through β), bronchial smooth muscle relaxation, glycogenolysis, calorigenesis, bladder and intestinal relaxation and increase in insulin secretion (through β_2 receptors).
- **Drugs** which **block** α receptors are phenoxybenzamine, pentalamine and yohimbine.
- β blockers are, propanolol, proctolol and Butoxamine.
- Sympathetic nervous system is called for action only in **emergencies, stressful** conditions preparing animal to **fight** or **run away** in order to protect itself.
- The preganglionic **parasympathetic** fibres travelling in the IX cranial nerve are contributed by inferior **salivatory** nucleus.
- **Occipital** region of the cerebral cortex is most likely region involved in pre-epileptic scintillation **aura**.
- **Nicotinic** receptors of **Ach** are involved in **excitatory** transmission in **autonomic** ganglia.
- This nicotinic transmission can be blocked by **curare**.
- The **fall** of BP during **flexadilisation** (I/V injection of curare) for muscle relaxation during anaesthesia is due to its **blockade** of excitatory **nicotinic** transmission in sympathetic ganglia.

Chapter Fifteen

Regulation of Body Temperature

- **Core temperature** i.e. surrounding the **internal organs**, is **closely regulated**.
- The **skin temperature** can fluctuate by **20 C°** on either side of the normal **core value** (37 C° or so).
- The **hypothalamus** acts as a **thermostat** of the body. It receives **inputs** from **thermoreceptors** and initiates appropriate heat **conserving** or loss **mechanisms**.
- **Increased blood flow** to the skin (as happens in summer) **brings warm blood** closer to the surface, **allowing more** heat to be **lost by radiation**, **conduction** and **convection**.
- In a **temperate climate**, more **than half** of the **heat loss** from the body occurs by **radiation.**
- **Neonates** can **raise** their **BMR** more effectively than adults, **largely** through metabolism of brown fat.
- Hence **non-shivering thermogenesis** is **more efficient** in **neonates** than in **adults**.
- **Sweating** is **controlled** by the **sympathetic** nervous system.
- **Skin temperature** is **usually lower** than **core temperature**.
- **During profuse sweating** (as happens during exposure to hot environment) **fluid** and **salts** are **lost** from the body in **large amounts.**
- This can **lead** to variety of symptoms **collectively called** as **heat exhaustion**.

- In **humid conditions,** sweat evaporates **more slowly** and is therefore less effective means of heat loss.
- **Thyroid hormones** stimulate **oxidative metabolism** and **generate heat**.
- Hence **secretion** of thyroid hormone is **enhanced** during **prolonged exposure** to **cold.**
- **Sweat rates rise** progressively during the **initial weeks** of **acclimatization** to high **ambient temperature.**
- **Aldosterone** secretion is **increased.** This leads to increased reabsorption of **salt from the urine and sweat and** fall in **sweat's salt content.**
- As the **sweat rate increases,** the body will lose **water. ADH will** be **increased** and urine output **will fall.**
- Hence a **person moving** from **temperate to tropical** area will show excessive **sweating, reduced salt** in **sweat** and less **urine production.**

Chapter Sixteen

Stress Syndrome

- **Classic** response to **stress**, whether psychological or physical is the **increased** secretion of **cortisol** from **adrenal cortex** and activation of **sympathetic** nervous system, including release of **epinephrine** from adrenal **medulla.**
- The **function** of these responses is to **prepare** individual for **fight** or **flight** and for **coping** with new situation.
- Other **hormones** released during **stress** include **aldosterone**, **vasopressin**, **glucagon**, **growth hormone** and **prolactin**. Insulin secretion is usually decreased.